DASH DIET 2025

110 Recipes New Eating Strategies for a Healthy Life A Modern Approach to Health and Wellbeing

KLARLOCK

DISCLAIMER

This book aims to provide useful and informative material on the topics covered in the publication. It is sold with the understanding that the author and publisher are not engaged in rendering any personal medical, health care, or other professional services in the book. The reader should consult his or her physician, health care provider, or other competent professional before adopting any suggestions in this book or drawing any conclusions. The author and publisher expressly disclaim responsibility for any liability, loss, or risk, personal or otherwise, arising, directly or indirectly, from the use and application of any contents of this book.

NOTE

All the recipes in this book are designed for four people. For this quantity, the ingredients indicated in the recipes must be considered. If you need to change the portion, it is recommended to proportionally adjust the doses of the ingredients. It is also recommended to carefully follow the preparation and cooking instructions to obtain the best result. In the context of this book, when we refer to "a cup" as a unit of measurement for ingredients, we mean using a standard kitchen cup with a capacity of approximately 240 milliliters. It is essential to use a measuring cup to get the right quantities of ingredients. If you don't have a measuring cup, you can use a graduated measuring cup, making sure to correctly correspond to the proportions indicated. Here are some examples 1 Cup of flour 100 gr. 1 cup of rice 200 gr. 1 Cup of Quinoa 200 gr

TABLE OF CONTENT

RECIPES FIRST DISHES

RECIPES SECOND DISHES

218 ASPARAGUS AND RICOTTA PIE

220 GRATINATED CAULIFLOWER WITH TOMATO AND BASIL SAUCE

222 ROMAN-STYLE ARTICHOKES WITH POTATOES

224 BAKED ASPARAGUS WITH HAM AND CHEESE

226 ASPARAGUS AND BACON OMELETTE

228 SLICED BEEF WITH ARUGULA AND TOMATOES

230 BEEF STEW WITH POTATOES AND CARROTS

233 BEEF AND ASPARAGUS IN A PAN

235 ROAST BEEF WITH ARTICHOKES AND POTATOES

237 BEEF MEATBALLS WITH SPINACH

240 PORK CHOPS WITH APPLES AND POTATOES

243 ROAST PORK WITH PLUM AND CARROTS

SIDE DISH RECIPES

INTRODUCTION TO THE DASH DIET

The Diet Dash 2025 (Dietary Approaches to Stop Hypertension) is a dietary regime created by the United States National Institute for Health (NIH) with the aim of preventing or improving hypertension (high blood pressure). Based on scientific research, the DASH diet aims to lower blood pressure through a dietary approach rich in specific nutrients and with a reduced sodium content. What makes the DASH diet special? Emphasis on fruits, vegetables and whole grains: These foods are rich in potassium, magnesium, calcium and fiber, all nutrients that help regulate blood pressure. Lean protein: The DASH diet encourages consumption of protein from sources such as fish, poultry, legumes and tofu, which provide essential nutrients without increasing saturated cholesterol levels. Low-fat dairy products:

Choosing dairy products like skim milk or low-fat yogurt provides calcium and vitamin D important for bone health, without excess saturated fat. Healthy Fats: The DASH diet emphasizes monounsaturated and polyunsaturated fats from sources like olive oil, avocados and nuts, which support heart health. Reduce sodium: Excessive sodium consumption can increase blood pressure. The DASH diet limits sodium intake to less than 2,300 milligrams per day (or 1,500 milligrams for specific categories of people). Limiting Added Sugars: Excessive consumption of added sugars can lead to weight gain and other health problems. The DASH diet encourages limiting added sugars, favoring fresh, whole foods.

If you're interested in trying the DASH diet, here are some tips to get you started: Consult your doctor: Before making any significant changes to your diet, it's important to talk to your doctor to make sure it's right for you, especially if you have pre-existing medical conditions . Start Gradually: You don't need to suddenly upend your eating habits. Start with small changes, like adding more fruits and vegetables to your meals or choosing whole grains instead of refined ones.

THE HISTORY AND ORIGIN OF THE DASH DIET

The DASH diet (Dietary Approaches to Stop Hypertension) was born in the early 1980s at the National Institutes of Health of the United States (NIH) with the aim of finding a nutritional approach capable of lowering blood pressure effectively and Safe. The research conducted by NIH doctors and researchers was based on the observation of several populations that had significantly lower rates of hypertension than Western countries. By analyzing their eating habits, a common characteristic was identified: a high consumption of fruit, vegetables, whole grains and low-fat dairy products, associated with a low intake of sodium and saturated fat. These observations led to the creation of the DASH diet, officially presented in 1997 as a diet capable of preventing and improving hypertension in

natural and complementary way to the use of drugs. Factors that contributed to the development of the DASH diet: Concern about hypertension: Hypertension was a growing public health problem, with a significant impact on morbidity and mortality. A non-pharmacological approach to its management was sought. Research on nutrition and blood pressure: Epidemiological and experimental studies had already highlighted the role of some nutrients and dietary patterns in the control of blood pressure.

Comparison between food cultures: The analysis of the eating habits of populations with low rates of hypertension has provided important insights for the definition of the key principles of the DASH diet.

Evolution of the DASH diet over time: Over the years, the DASH diet has been the subject of further research and refinement, with the addition of new recommendations and adaptation to the specific nutritional needs of different age groups and health conditions.

Today, the DASH diet is recognized as an effective and safe dietary approach for preventing and controlling hypertension, as well as promoting better overall health. It is recommended by numerous health authorities and medical associations around the world. The DASH diet represents an example of how nutrition can play a fundamental role in managing health and preventing chronic diseases.

WHAT IS THE DASH DIET

The DASH diet is a type of diet developed to help prevent and control high blood pressure. This diet is based on increasing your intake of nutrient-rich foods known to have a positive effect on blood pressure, such as fruits, vegetables, whole grains, lean proteins, and low-fat dairy products. In particular, the DASH diet involves a high consumption of potassium, magnesium, calcium, fiber and plant proteins. The DASH diet also involves reducing your intake of foods high in saturated fat, cholesterol, and sodium, which are known to increase the risk of hypertension.

Foods such as red meats, sugary drinks, fried foods, and processed foods are limited on the DASH diet. The main goal of the DASH diet is to increase the intake of healthy nutrients and reduce the intake of harmful substances. Numerous studies have shown that the DASH diet can help lower blood pressure and improve overall heart and blood vessel health. In summary, the DASH diet is a healthy, balanced diet that can help prevent and control high blood pressure. It promotes a high consumption of nutritious foods and a reduction in the intake of substances harmful to health, which can lead to numerous benefits for the overall health of the heart and blood vessels.

THE BENEFITS OF THE DASH DIET

The DASH diet was initially developed to help people with high blood pressure, but has since been shown to have a wide range of health benefits. One of the main benefits of the DASH diet is its ability to reduce the risk of heart disease and stroke. That's because the diet emphasizes foods that are low in saturated fat and rich in nutrients known to be heart-healthy, such as potassium, magnesium and fiber. Studies have shown that people who follow the DASH diet have lower blood pressure and lower levels of LDL (or "bad") cholesterol, which are two key risk factors for heart disease and stroke. Helps with weight loss and weight management The DASH diet is also effective for weight loss and weight management. Because the diet emphasizes whole, nutrient-rich foods and limits processed foods and sugary drinks can help people reduce overall calorie intake without feeling hungry or deprived. Studies have shown that people who follow the DASH diet lose weight and are more easily able to maintain weight over time. Reduces the risk of some types of cancer, research has also shown that the DASH diet may reduce the risk of some types of cancer, including colorectal, breast and prostate cancer. That's because the diet emphasizes foods rich in antioxidants and other nutrients that have been shown to have anticancer properties. Additionally, the DASH diet encourages consumption of foods rich in fiber, which can help promote regular bowel movements and reduce the risk of colon cancer.

Sustainable and easy to follow Finally, one of the main benefits of the DASH diet is that it is sustainable and easy to follow. Unlike many fad diets that require strict adherence to complex rules and restrictions, the DASH diet is a flexible, adaptable eating plan that can be customized to suit individual tastes and preferences. This makes it more likely that people will stick to the diet long-term, which can lead to long-lasting health benefits. The DASH diet is a healthy eating plan that can provide a wide range of benefits to people of all ages and backgrounds. Whether you're looking to reduce your risk of heart disease, manage your weight, or just feel better overall, the DASH diet is a great place to start.

FUNDAMENTALS OF THE DASH DIET

The DASH (Dietary Approaches to Stop Hypertension) diet is based on solid nutritional principles that aim to reduce blood pressure naturally and safely, while promoting better overall health.

Here are the fundamental cornerstones of the DASH diet:

1. Abundant consumption of fruit and vegetables:

Recommended at least 810 servings per day.

Choose a variety of colors to get a broad spectrum of nutrients and antioxidants.

Choose fresh seasonal fruit and vegetables.

2. Whole grains as the basis of the diet:

Take 68 servings per day.

Opt for whole grains such as wholemeal bread, brown rice, wholemeal pasta and oats.

Whole grains provide fiber, vitamins, minerals and a prolonged sense of satiety.

3. Low-fat dairy products:

Include 23 servings per day.

Choose skim milk, low-fat yogurt or low-fat cheeses.

Dairy products provide calcium, vitamin D and proteins that are important for bone and muscle health.

4. Lean protein as your primary protein source: Eat 23 servings per day.

Opt for lean proteins such as fish, poultry, legumes, tofu and beans.

Lean proteins provide essential amino acids for building and maintaining tissue, without increasing saturated cholesterol levels.

5. Healthy Fats in Moderation:

Limit saturated and trans fats to less than 6 percent of total calories.

Focus on monounsaturated and polyunsaturated fats from sources such as olive oil, avocado, nuts and seeds.

Healthy fats promote heart health and reduce the risk of chronic diseases.

6. Reduce Sodium:

Limit sodium intake to less than 2,300 milligrams per day (or 1,500 milligrams for specific categories of people).

Reduce consumption of packaged, salted and processed foods.

Use herbs and spices to flavor dishes instead of salt.

EXAMPLES OF WEEKLY MENU

Here is an example of a weekly menu that follows the principles of the DASH diet:

Day 1:

Breakfast: Oat flakes with berries and nuts, low-fat yogurt with fresh fruit.

Lunch: Quinoa salad with grilled vegetables and grilled chicken, wholemeal bread.

Snack: Fresh fruit, raw vegetables with hummus.

Dinner: Baked salmon with grilled vegetables.

Day 2:

Breakfast: Fruit smoothie with low-fat yogurt and chia seeds, toasted wholemeal bread with avocado.

Lunch: Lentil soup with wholemeal bread, green salad with tomatoes and cucumbers.

Snack: Mix of dried fruit and nuts, low-fat yogurt.

Dinner: Sautéed tofu with vegetables and brown rice.

Day 3:

Breakfast: Scrambled eggs with vegetables and wholemeal bread, low-fat yogurt with fresh fruit.

Lunch: Chickpea salad with tuna, tomatoes, olives and low-fat feta, wholemeal bread.

Snack: Fresh fruit, raw vegetables with hummus.

Dinner: Baked chicken with sweet potatoes and steamed broccoli.

Day 4:

Breakfast: Omelette with vegetables and cheese

low fat, wholemeal toast with avocado.

Lunch: Quinoa salad with grilled vegetables and grilled tempeh, wholemeal bread.

Snack: Low-fat yogurt with fresh fruit and granola.

Dinner: Baked salmon with sweet potatoes and steamed asparagus.

Day 5:

Breakfast: Fruit smoothie with low-fat yogurt and peanut butter, toasted wholemeal bread with almond butter.

Lunch: Minestrone soup with wholemeal bread, green salad with tomatoes and low-fat mozzarella.

Snack: Mix of dried fruit and nuts, low-fat yogurt.

Dinner: Sautéed tofu with vegetables and brown rice.

Day 6: Breakfast: Baked eggs with avocado and wholemeal bread, low-fat yogurt with fresh fruit.

Lunch: Chicken salad with avocado, tomatoes, cucumbers and low-fat feta, wholemeal bread.

Snack: Fresh fruit, raw vegetables with hummus.

Dinner: Baked salmon with sweet potatoes and steamed Brussels sprouts.

Day 7: Breakfast: Wholemeal pancakes with maple syrup and fresh fruit, low-fat yogurt with fresh fruit.

Lunch: Quinoa salad with grilled vegetables and grilled shrimp, wholemeal bread.

Snack: Fresh fruit, raw vegetables with hummus.

Dinner: Baked chicken with sweet potatoes and steamed carrots.

PHYSICAL ACTIVITY AND DASH DIET

Combine physical activity and the DASH diet for optimal health

The DASH diet, rich in fruits, vegetables, whole grains, lean proteins and low-fat dairy products, is an effective dietary approach for the prevention and control of hypertension. However, to maximize health benefits and achieve overall well-being, combining the DASH diet with regular physical activity is essential.

Why is physical activity important on the DASH diet?

Enhances the blood pressure lowering effect: Physical exercise contributes to reducing blood pressure independently of diet, acting on different physiological mechanisms.

Promotes weight control: Combined with a healthy diet such as DASH, physical activity helps

to maintain a healthy body weight or lose it gradually, reducing the risk of obesity and its complications.

Improves Cardiovascular Health: Regular exercise strengthens the heart and lungs, increases endurance, and decreases the risk of heart disease, stroke, and type 2 diabetes.

Reduces Stress: Physical activity helps reduce stress levels, which can contribute to high blood pressure and other health problems.

Improves mood and quality of life: Regular exercise is associated with improved mood, energy levels and quality of sleep, contributing to greater overall well-being.

What types of physical activity are recommended on the DASH diet?

According to the American Physical Activity Guidelines, it is recommended that you do at least 150 minutes of moderate aerobic physical activity or 75 minutes of vigorous aerobic physical activity each week.

Moderate aerobic physical activity includes brisk walking, swimming, cycling, or dancing. Vigorous aerobic physical activity includes running, sprinting, or brisk swimming. In addition to aerobic physical activity, it is important to also include strength exercises at least two days a week. Strength exercises help build and maintain muscle mass, which in turn promotes a more efficient metabolism and burns more calories even at rest.

THE FUTURE OF THE DASH DIET PERSPECTIVES AND NEW RESEARCH

The DASH diet, with its strong scientific basis and proven health benefits, continues to enjoy great popularity and recognition as an effective dietary approach for preventing and controlling hypertension and promoting overall health. Looking to the future, several trends and new research are emerging in the DASH diet landscape, positioning it as an ever-evolving dietary model that is adaptable to changing nutritional needs:

1. Personalization and cultural adaptation:

Customizing the DASH diet to individual needs, cultural preferences, and specific health conditions is an area of growing interest.

Future research will focus on adapting the DASH diet to different cultural and demographic contexts, ensuring access and equity for all.

2. Integration with innovative technologies: The use of innovative technologies, such as smartphone apps, nutritional monitoring tools and telemedicine platforms, can facilitate meal planning, diet management and personalized support for those following the DASH diet.

3. Emphasis on gut health:

The connection between gut health and overall health is becoming more and more evident. Future research will explore the role of the DASH diet in promoting a healthy gut microbiome and its potential impact on chronic disease prevention.

RECIPES APPETIZERS AND SMOOTHIE

CHICKPEA AND TOMATO SALAD

Preparation time: 10 minutes

Doses for 4 people:

400g canned chickpeas, drained and rinsed

3 ripe tomatoes, cut into cubes

1/2 red onion, chopped

1/4 cup chopped fresh parsley

2 tablespoons fresh lemon juice

2 tablespoons extra virgin olive oil

Preparation:

In a large bowl, combine the chickpeas, diced tomatoes, chopped red onion and fresh parsley. In a cup, mix the lemon juice and extra virgin olive oil. Pour the vinaigrette over the bowl of chickpeas and tomatoes and mix well. Serve in individual portions.

TOMATO AND AVOCADO CROSTINI

Preparation time: 15 minutes

Doses for 4 people:

4 slices wholemeal bread, cut in half

1 ripe avocado, mashed

2 ripe tomatoes, cut into thin slices

1/4 cup chopped fresh herbs

(basil, parsley, thyme, etc.)

Preparation:

Toast the slices of wholemeal bread until golden brown. Spread the mashed avocado on the toasted bread slices. Place the tomato slices on top of the avocado. Sprinkle with chopped fresh herbs. Serve in portions of 2 croutons per person.

SMOKED SALMON ROLLUP

Preparation time: 10 minutes

Doses for 4 people:

8 slices of smoked salmon

250 g of light spreadable cheese

1 tablespoon fresh lemon juice

1/4 cup chopped red onion

1/4 cup chopped cucumbers

Preparation

In a bowl, mix the cream cheese, fresh lemon juice, chopped red onion and chopped cucumber. Arrange the salmon slices on a cutting board. Spread the cream cheese mixture over the salmon slices. Roll the salmon slices well, forming a roll. Cut the salmon roll into 8 pieces. Serve in portions of 2 pieces per person.

SHRIMP AND VEGETABLES SKEWERS

Preparation time: 20 minutes

Doses for 4 people:

16 large prawns, peeled and cleaned

1 red pepper, diced

1 yellow pepper, diced

1 red onion, diced

8 cherry tomatoes, halved

2 tablespoons extra virgin olive oil

2 tablespoons fresh lemon juice

1 clove garlic, finely chopped

1 teaspoon paprika

Preparation

In a bowl mix the extra virgin olive oil, fresh lemon juice, chopped garlic and paprika. Thread the prawns, peppers, onion and cherry tomatoes alternately onto 8 wooden skewers. Brush the skewers with olive oil and spice marinade. Grill the skewers on a hot grill for 810 minutes, turning them halfway through cooking. Serve hot.

EGGS STUFFED WITH HUMMUS

Preparation time: 15 minutes

Doses for 4 people:

8 hard boiled eggs

1/2 cup hummus

2 tablespoons Greek yogurt

2 tablespoons fresh lemon juice

1/4 teaspoon salt

1/4 teaspoon sweet paprika

Freshly ground black pepper, to taste

1 tablespoon chopped fresh parsley

Preparation

Cut the hard-boiled eggs in half and remove the yolks. In a bowl, mash the egg yolks with a fork and add the hummus, Greek yogurt, fresh lemon juice, salt and sweet paprika. Mix until you obtain a smooth and creamy mixture. Using a spoon, fill the egg halves with the hummus mixture. Sprinkle with freshly ground black pepper and chopped fresh parsley. Serve cold.

BLACK BEAN BRUSCHETTA

Preparation time: 20 minutes

Doses for 4 people:

4 slices of Tuscan or rustic bread

1 can black beans, drained and rinsed

1 ripe tomato, diced

1/4 cup chopped red onion

2 tablespoons chopped fresh coriander

1 tablespoon fresh lime juice

1/2 teaspoon ground cumin

Salt and freshly ground black pepper, to taste

1 peeled clove of garlic 2 tablespoons of extra virgin olive oil

Preparation

In a bowl, mix black beans, diced tomato, chopped red onion, chopped fresh cilantro, fresh lime juice, ground cumin, salt and freshly ground black pepper. Mix well to combine the ingredients. Grill the slices of Tuscan bread or rustic bread on a hot grill or on a hot griddle until they are lightly golden and crispy. Rub the garlic clove over each slice of grilled bread. Drizzle each slice of bread with a drizzle of extra virgin olive oil and then with a generous portion of the black bean mixture. Serve immediately as an appetizer or side dish.

COURGETTE CARPACCIO

**Preparation time:
approximately 1015 minutes**

Doses for: 24 people

Ingredients:

23 medium courgettes

Extra virgin olive oil

Salt and pepper to taste.

Lemon juice

Flaked parmesan

Fresh basil

Preparation

Cut the courgettes into thin slices with a potato peeler or mandolin. Arrange the slices on a serving plate. Season with extra virgin olive oil, salt, pepper and lemon juice. Add fresh basil leaves and parmesan flakes to taste. Serve immediately.

GUACAMOLE AND CORN CHIPS

Preparation time:

approximately 2025 minutes

Doses for: 4 people

Ingredients:

2 ripe avocados

1 lemon

1 clove of garlic

Salt and pepper to taste.

4 corn tortillas

Olive oil

Preparation

For the guacamole: Mash two ripe avocados with a fork in a bowl. Add the juice of half a lemon, a pinch of salt and pepper and a chopped clove of garlic. Mix all the ingredients well and season with salt and pepper to taste. For the corn chips: Cut the corn tortillas into triangles with a sharp knife. Arrange the triangles on a baking sheet and sprinkle with olive oil and salt. Cook in a preheated oven at 180°C for approximately 1012 minutes or until the potatoes are golden and crispy. Serve the guacamole in a bowl with the hot corn chips on the side.

AUBERGINES CAPRESE

Preparation time: approximately 30 minutes

Servings: 46 people

Ingredients:

2 large aubergines

Salt and black pepper to taste

1/2 cup all-purpose flour

3 eggs

1/4 cup vegetable oil

46 large slices of fresh mozzarella

46 large slices of ripe tomato

Fresh basil leaves

Balsamic vinegar (optional)

Preparation

Preheat the oven to 190°C. Cut the eggplant into 1/2-inch-thick rounds and sprinkle with salt. Let them sit for 1015 minutes, then rinse and pat dry with paper towels. Place the flour in a shallow dish and season with salt and black pepper. Beat the eggs in a separate shallow dish. Dip each slice of aubergine in the flour, then in the beaten eggs and shake off the excess. Heat vegetable oil in a large skillet over medium-high heat. Add the eggplant slices and cook until golden brown on both sides, about 23 minutes per side. Transfer the aubergine slices onto a baking tray lined with baking paper. Top each slice with a slice of mozzarella and a slice of tomato. Bake for 1015 minutes until cheese is melted and bubbly. Garnish with fresh basil leaves and a drizzle of balsamic vinegar, if desired. Serve hot.

VEGETABLE OMELET FLADS

Preparation time:

about 20 minutes

Servings: 24 people

Ingredients:

6 large eggs

1/4 cup milk

Salt and black pepper to taste

1 tablespoon olive oil

1 small onion, diced

1 bell pepper, diced

1 small courgette, diced

1 small yellow squash, diced

1/4 cup shredded cheddar cheese

Preparation

Whisk together the eggs, milk, salt, and black pepper in a medium bowl. Heat the olive oil in a large skillet over medium-high heat. Add the onion, bell pepper, zucchini, yellow squash and sauté until tender, about 57 minutes. Pour the egg mixture over the vegetables and cook until set, about 57 minutes. Sprinkle the shredded cheddar cheese over the omelette and let it melt. A spatula folds the omelette in half and slides it onto a serving plate. Serve hot, garnished with fresh herbs or chopped tomatoes, if desired

STRAWBERRY AND BANANA SMOOTHIE

Preparation time: 5 minutes

Servings: 1

Ingredients:

1 banana

1 cup fresh strawberries

1/2 cup skim milk

1/2 cup low-fat Greek yogurt

1 tablespoon honey

Preparation

Add all ingredients to a blender and blend until smooth. Serve immediately.

SPINACH AND BANANA SMOOTHIE

Preparation time: 5 minutes

Servings: 1

Ingredients:

2 cups fresh spinach

1 banana

1/2 cup skim milk

1/2 cup low-fat yogurt

1 tablespoon honey

Preparation

Add all ingredients to a blender and blend until smooth. Serve immediately. If you want a thinner consistency, you can add more milk. If you prefer a thicker consistency, you can add more yogurt.

BLUEBERRY AND ALMONDS SMOOTHIE

Preparation time: 5 minutes

Servings: 1

ingredients

1 cup fresh blueberries

1/2 cup unsweetened almond milk

1/2 cup low-fat Greek yogurt

1/4 cup almonds

1 tablespoon honey

Preparation

Add all ingredients to a blender and blend until smooth. Serve immediately.

KIWI AND BANANA SMOOTHIE

Preparation time: 5 minutes

Servings: 1

ingredients

2 kiwis

1 banana

1/2 cup low-fat Greek yogurt

1/2 cup skim milk

1 tablespoon honey

Preparation

Add all ingredients to a blender and blend until smooth. Serve immediately. If you want a thinner consistency, you can add more milk. If you prefer a thicker consistency, you can add more yogurt.

MANGO AND PINEAPPLE SMOOTHIES

Preparation time: 5 minutes

Servings: 1

ingredients

1 cup fresh or frozen mango chunks

1 cup fresh or frozen pineapple chunks

1/2 cup low-fat Greek yogurt

1/2 cup unsweetened almond milk

1 tablespoon honey

Preparation

Add all ingredients to a blender and blend until smooth. Serve immediately.

AVOCADO AND CILANTRO SMOOTHIE

Preparation time: 5 minutes

Servings: 1

ingredients

1/2 avocado

1 cup fresh spinach

1/2 cup fresh cilantro

1/2 cup unsweetened almond milk

1/2 cup low-fat Greek yogurt

1/4 teaspoon ground cumin

1/4 teaspoon salt

Preparation

Add all ingredients to a blender and blend until smooth. Serve immediately. If you want a thinner consistency, you can add more milk. If you prefer a thicker consistency, you can add more yogurt.

STRAWBERRY AND RHUBARB SMOOTHIE

Preparation time: 5 minutes

Servings: 1

ingredients

1 cup fresh strawberries

1/2 cup fresh rhubarb, chopped

1/2 cup low-fat Greek yogurt

1/2 cup unsweetened almond milk

1 tablespoon honey

Preparation

Add all ingredients to a blender and blend until smooth. Serve immediately.

PEACH AND MANGO SMOOTHIE

Preparation time: 5 minutes

Servings: 1

Ingredients:

1 cup fresh or frozen mango chunks

1 peach, pitted and chopped

1/2 cup low-fat Greek yogurt

1/2 cup unsweetened almond milk

1 tablespoon honey

Preparation

Add all ingredients to a blender and blend until smooth, serve immediately.

BANANA AND COCONUT SMOOTHIE

65

Preparation time: 5 minutes

Servings: 1

ingredients

1 banana

1/2 cup coconut milk

1/2 cup low-fat Greek yogurt

1/2 cup unsweetened almond milk

1 tablespoon honey

Preparation

Add all ingredients to a blender and blend until smooth. Serve immediately.

STRAWBERRY AND VANILLA YOGURT SMOOTHIE

Preparation time: 5 minutes

Servings: 1

ingredients

1 cup fresh strawberries

1/2 cup low-fat Greek yogurt

1/2 cup unsweetened almond milk

1 tablespoon honey

1/2 teaspoon vanilla extract

Preparation

Add all ingredients to a blender and blend until smooth. Serve immediately.

RECIPES
FIRST DISHES

SPAGHETTI WITH ARTICHOKES

Preparation time: 30 minutes.

serving 4 people

Ingredients:

500 grams of spaghetti

2 cans (140 g each) of artichokes

hearts, drained and quartered

3 cloves garlic, minced

1/4 cup olive oil

1/4 cup freshly grated parmesan

1/4 cup chopped fresh parsley

Salt and pepper to taste

Preparation

Cook the spaghetti in a large pot of boiling salted water according to package directions, until al dente. Drain the spaghetti, reserving 1/2 cup of the pasta water. While the spaghetti cooks, heat the olive oil in a large skillet over medium heat. Add the garlic and cook for 1/2 minute, until fragrant. Add the artichoke hearts to the pan and cook for 3 to 4 minutes, until lightly browned. Add the cooked spaghetti to the pan with the artichokes and stir to combine. If the pasta seems dry, add a little of the reserved pasta water. Remove the pan from the heat and stir in the parmesan and parsley. Season with salt and pepper to taste. Serve the spaghetti with artichokes immediately, garnished with more parmesan and parsley if desired. Enjoy your meal.

SPAGHETTI WITH SEAFOOD

Preparation time: 45 minutes.

serving 4 people.

Ingredients:

1 500 g of spaghetti

1 pound mixed seafood (e.g

such as prawns, scallops and calamari),

clean and gutted

3 cloves garlic, minced

1/4 cup olive oil

1/2 glass of dry white wine

1 (28-ounce) can diced tomatoes, drained

1/4 teaspoon red pepper flakes

Salt and pepper to taste

1/4 cup chopped fresh parsley

Lemon wedges, to serve

Preparation

Cook the spaghetti in a large pot of boiling salted water according to package directions, until al dente. Drain the spaghetti, reserving 1/2 cup of the pasta water. While the spaghetti cooks, heat the olive oil in a large skillet over medium heat. Add the garlic and cook for 1/2 minute, until fragrant. Add the mixed seafood to the pan and cook for 3 to 4 minutes, until cooked through. Remove the seafood from the pan and set aside.

Add the white wine to the pan and bring it to a boil. Cook for 1/2 minutes, until the wine has reduced by half. Add the diced tomatoes and chili flakes to the pan and bring to a simmer. Cook for 5/7 minutes, until the sauce has thickened slightly. Return seafood to pan and toss to coat with sauce. Season with salt and pepper to taste. Add the cooked spaghetti to the pan with the seafood and stir to combine. If the pasta seems dry, add a little of the reserved pasta water. Remove the pan from the heat and add the chopped parsley. Serve the spaghetti with seafood immediately, garnished with lemon wedges. Enjoy your meal.

SPAGHETTI WITH PUMPKIN WITH MARINARA SAUCE AND PARMESAN

Preparation time:

about 45 minutes.

for 4 people:

Ingredients:

1/2 kg spaghetti

500 g of pumpkin,

peeled and cut into cubes

1 onion, chopped

2 cloves garlic, minced

1/4 cup olive oil

2 cups marinara sauce

1/2 cup grated parmesan,

plus more for garnish

Salt and pepper to taste

Fresh basil for garnish

Preparation

Preheat the oven to 190°C (190°F). Line a baking tray with baking paper and arrange the pumpkin in a single layer. Cook for about 20/25 minutes, until the pumpkin is soft and lightly golden. Remove the pumpkin from the oven and set it aside. In a large saucepan, bring plenty of salted water to the boil. Cook the spaghetti al dente, following the instructions on the package. Drain and set aside. In a large skillet, heat the olive oil over medium heat. Add the onion and garlic and cook until soft and golden, about 5 to 7 minutes.

Add the marinara sauce and squash to the pan and mix well. Simmer for about 5 minutes, until the sauce is hot and the squash is fully incorporated. Add the spaghetti to the pan and toss well to coat with the sauce. Add the grated parmesan and mix again to melt it. Season with salt and pepper to taste. Serve the spaghetti squash with marinara sauce and parmesan hot, garnished with additional grated parmesan and fresh basil. Enjoy your meal.

BROWN RICE PASTA WITH BLACK CABBAGE AND WALNUT PESTO

Preparation time:

about 30 minutes.

for 4 people:

Ingredients:

400 g brown rice pasta

1 cabbage, washed and chopped

1/2 cup walnuts, toasted and chopped

1/2 cup grated parmesan

2 cloves garlic, minced

1/2 cup olive oil

Salt and pepper to taste.

Preparation

In a large saucepan, bring plenty of salted water to the boil. Cook the brown rice pasta al dente, following the instructions on the package. Drain and set aside. In a large skillet, heat the olive oil over medium heat. Add the cabbage and cook until soft, about 5 to 7 minutes. Add the nuts and garlic to the pan and cook for a further 2 to 3 minutes, stirring often. Transfer the cabbage, walnuts, and garlic to a blender or food processor. Add the grated parmesan and a pinch of salt and pepper. Blend all the ingredients until you obtain a smooth pesto. Add the kale pesto to the brown rice pasta and mix well to cover all the pasta with the pesto. Season with salt and pepper to taste. Serve the brown rice pasta with hot kale and walnut pesto. Enjoy your meal!

LINGUINE WITH PRAWNS, SPINACH AND TOMATOES

Preparation time:

about 30 minutes.

for 4 people:

Ingredients:

400 g of linguine

400 g of peeled and cleaned prawns

200g cherry tomatoes, cut in half

200g of fresh spinach

4 cloves of garlic minced

1/2 cup olive oil

1/2 glass of white wine

Salt and pepper to taste

Preparation

In a large saucepan, bring plenty of salted water to the boil. Cook the linguine al dente, following the instructions on the package. Drain and set aside. In a large skillet, heat the olive oil over medium-high heat. Add the garlic and cook until browned, about 1 to 2 minutes. Add the prawns to the pan and cook for 2 to 3 minutes, until pink. Remove the prawns from the pan and set aside. Add the white wine to the pan and cook until reduced by half, about 2 to 3 minutes.

Add the cherry tomatoes and cook for 2/3 minutes, until soft. Add the spinach to the pan and cook for 1/2 minute, until wilted. Add the shrimp to the pan and stir well to heat through. Add the linguine to the pan and mix well to cover all the pasta with the shrimp and vegetable sauce. Season with salt and pepper to taste. Serve the linguine with prawns, spinach and cherry tomatoes piping hot. Enjoy your meal!

TOMATO SOUP AND VEGETABLES WITH QUINOA

Preparation time:

about 45/50 minutes.

for 4 people

ingredients

2 tablespoons of olive oil

1 onion, chopped

2 cloves garlic, minced

2 carrots, diced

2 stalks celery, diced

1 red pepper, diced

1 can of whole tomatoes

1 liter of vegetable broth

1/2 cup quinoa

1 teaspoon dried oregano

Salt and pepper to taste

Chopped fresh parsley (for garnish)

Preparation

In a large pot, heat the olive oil over medium heat. Add the onion and garlic and cook until golden brown, about 2 to 3 minutes. Add the carrots, celery and pepper to the pot and cook for 5/7 minutes, until the vegetables are soft. Add the can of tomatoes and vegetable broth to the pot and bring to a boil. Reduce heat and simmer for 15/20 minutes. Add the quinoa and oregano to the pot and continue to cook for another 15 to 20 minutes, or until the quinoa is cooked. Season with salt and pepper to taste. Serve the tomato and vegetable soup with the quinoa piping hot, garnished with chopped fresh parsley.

SLOW COOKING

VEGETABLE SOUP

WITH BARLEY

Preparation time:

about 10/15 minutes for preparation,

6/8 hours for the slow cooker.

(for 4/6 people):

ingredients

2 tablespoons of olive oil

1 onion, chopped

2 cloves garlic, minced

2 carrots, diced

2 stalks celery, diced

2 potatoes, diced

1 cup pearl barley

1 can of cannellini beans,
rinsed and drained

1 liter vegetable broth

1 cup diced tomatoes

1 teaspoon dried thyme

Salt and pepper to taste

Chopped fresh parsley (for garnish)

Preparation:

In a large skillet, heat the olive oil over medium heat. Add the onion and garlic and cook until golden brown, about 2 to 3 minutes. Transfer the onion and garlic to the slow cooker. Add the carrots, celery and potatoes and mix well.

Add pearl barley, cannellini beans, vegetable broth, diced tomatoes, and dried thyme to the slow cooker. Mix well. Cover the pot and simmer for 6 to 8 hours, or until the vegetables and barley are soft and cooked. Season with salt and pepper to taste. Serve the slow-cooked vegetable soup with hot orzo, garnished with chopped fresh parsley.

**PUMPKIN SOUP WITH
HONEY AND GINGER**

Preparation time: approximately 20 minutes.

(for 4/6 people):

ingredients

1 kg of pumpkin, peeled and cut into cubes

2 apples, peeled and cut into cubes

1 onion, chopped

2 cloves garlic, minced

1 piece of fresh ginger, peeled and grated

1 liter of vegetable broth

1/2 cup fresh cream

2 tablespoons butter

1 teaspoon ground cinnamon

Salt and pepper to taste

toasted pumpkin seeds (for garnish)

Preparation

In a large saucepan, melt the butter over medium heat. Add the onion and garlic and cook until golden brown, about 2 to 3 minutes. Add the pumpkin, apples and grated ginger to the pot and mix well. Add the vegetable broth, ground cinnamon, salt and pepper to the pot and mix well. Bring everything to the boil and then lower the heat. Cover the pot and simmer for 25 to 30 minutes, or until the squash and apples are soft. Blend the soup with an immersion blender until you obtain a smooth and homogeneous cream. Add fresh cream to the soup and mix well. Serve the pumpkin soup with apples and hot ginger, garnished with toasted pumpkin seeds.

CHICKPEA AND VEGETABLE SOUP

Preparation time:

approximately 1 hour and 30 minutes.

(for 4 people):

ingredients

1 cup dried chickpeas

2 carrots, peeled and diced

2 sticks of celery, diced

1 onion, chopped

2 cloves garlic, minced

1 liter of vegetable broth

1 can of peeled tomatoes

1 teaspoon cumin powder

1 teaspoon coriander powder

1/2 teaspoon chili powder

Salt and pepper to taste

Chopped fresh parsley (for garnish)

Preparation

The night before, soak the dried chickpeas in a bowl covered with water. Leave them to soak overnight. The next day, drain the chickpeas and rinse them well under running water. In a large pot, sauté the onion and garlic over medium heat. Add the carrots and celery and cook for another 5 minutes. Add the dried chickpeas to the pot and cover with the vegetable broth. Add the peeled tomatoes, cumin, coriander, chilli powder, add salt and pepper to the pan and mix well. Bring everything to the boil and then lower the heat. Cover the pot and simmer for about 1 hour, or until the chickpeas are soft. Blend part of the soup with an immersion blender until smooth and creamy. Add fresh vegetables to the soup and cook for another 10 minutes. Serve the chickpea and vegetable soup hot, garnished with chopped fresh parsley.

BROCCOLI AND CHEESE SOUP

Preparation time:

about 30/40 minutes.

(for 4 people):

ingredients

2 broccoli, chopped

1 onion, chopped

2 cloves garlic, minced

1 liter of vegetable broth

1 cup of milk

1/2 cup cheddar cheese, shredded

1/4 grated parmesan

2 tablespoons butter

Salt and pepper to taste.

Preparation

In a large pot, sauté the onion and garlic in the butter over medium heat. Add the broccoli to the pot and cook for 5 minutes, stirring occasionally. Add the vegetable broth to the pan and bring it to the boil. Reduce the heat and cover the pan. Simmer for 15 to 20 minutes or until broccoli is tender. Blend the soup with an immersion blender until you obtain a smooth and homogeneous cream. Add the milk and cheese to the pot and mix well. Continue to cook the soup over medium/low heat, stirring often, until the cheese is completely melted. Season with salt and pepper to taste. Serve the broccoli and cheese soup hot, garnished with a sprinkling of grated parmesan.

QUINOA AND BLACK BEANS SALAD

Preparation time:

approximately 30 minutes

(for 4 people):

ingredients

1 cup quinoa, rinsed and drained

2 cups of water

1 can black beans, rinsed and drained

1 red pepper, diced

1/2 red onion, diced

1/2 cup sweet corn

1 ripe avocado, diced

1/4 cup fresh cilantro, chopped

2 tablespoons of olive oil

2 tablespoons lime juice

Salt and pepper to taste.

Preparation

In a medium saucepan, bring the water and quinoa to a boil. Reduce the heat, cover the pot and cook for about 15 minutes or until the quinoa is soft and the water has been absorbed. Remove the pan from the heat and leave to cool for a few minutes. In a large bowl, combine the black beans, sweet pepper, onion, corn, avocado and cilantro. Mix well. Add the cooled quinoa to the bowl with the other ingredients and mix well. Add the olive oil and lime juice to the bowl and mix well to dress the salad. Season with salt and pepper to taste. Let the quinoa and black bean salad rest in the refrigerator for at least 30 minutes before serving.

BROWN RICE AND PAN-SAUTE VEGETABLES

Preparation time 10 minutes

Cooking time 20/25 minutes

(for 4 people)

ingredients

2 cups brown rice

4 cups of water

1 tablespoon olive oil

1 onion, diced

2 carrots, diced

2 courgettes, diced

1 red pepper, diced

1 clove garlic, minced

Salt and pepper to taste.

Preparation

In a medium saucepan, bring the water and brown rice to a boil. Reduce the heat, cover the pot and cook for about 20/25 minutes or until the rice is cooked and the water has been absorbed. Remove the pan from the heat and let the rice rest for a few minutes. In a large skillet, heat the olive oil over medium-high heat. Add the onion and cook for about 2/3 minutes or until soft and translucent. Add the carrots and cook for a further 2/3 minutes or until the carrots are soft. Add the courgettes, bell pepper and garlic to the pan and cook for about 5 to 7 minutes or until the vegetables are tender. Add the brown rice to the pan with the vegetables and stir well to combine the ingredients. Season with salt and pepper to taste. Serve hot as a side dish or main course.

WILD RICE AND MUSHROOMS PILAF

Preparation time:

approximately 1 hour and 15 minutes.

(for 4 people):

ingredients

1 cup wild rice

2 cups vegetable broth

1 tablespoon olive oil

1 onion, diced

2 cloves garlic, minced

8 ounces mixed mushrooms

(champignons, shiitake), thinly sliced

Salt and pepper to taste

Fresh parsley, chopped (optional)

Preparation

In a medium saucepan, bring the vegetable broth to a boil. Add the wild rice, cover the pot and reduce the heat. Cook for approximately 4550 minutes or until the rice is cooked and the water has been absorbed. Remove the pan from the heat and let the rice rest for a few minutes. In a skillet, heat the olive oil over medium-high heat. Add the onion and cook for about 23 minutes or until soft and translucent. Add the garlic and mushrooms to the pan and cook for about 57 minutes or until the mushrooms are soft and golden. Add the wild rice to the pan with the mushrooms and stir well to combine the ingredients. Season with salt and pepper to taste. Serve hot as a side dish or main course. Garnish with chopped fresh parsley, if desired.

CHICKEN AND VEGETABLE JAMBALAYA

Preparation time

approximately 45/60 minutes.

For 4 people

Ingredients:

500g diced chicken breast

1 onion chopped

2 cloves garlic, minced

1 diced green pepper

1 diced red pepper

1 stalk of celery chopped

2 cups rice

4 cups chicken broth

2 teaspoons of paprika

1 teaspoon cumin

1 teaspoon oregano

1 teaspoon thyme

1 teaspoon of salt

1/2 teaspoon black pepper

2 tablespoons vegetable oil

1 cup peeled tomatoes

Preparation

In a large pan, heat the oil and add the onion and garlic, fry until translucent. Add the chicken and cook until browned.

Add the peppers and celery and cook for 5/7
minutes, until tender. Add the rice and spices
(paprika, cumin, oregano, thyme, salt and
black pepper) and mix well. Add the chicken
broth and peeled tomatoes, stir and bring to
the boil. Lower the heat, cover and cook for
20/25 minutes, until the rice is cooked and the
liquid absorbed. Remove from the heat and let
rest for 5/10 minutes before serving. Enjoy
your meal!

FRIED RICE WITH
SHRIMP AND VEGETABLES

Preparation time: 40 minutes

Serves: 4 people

ingredients

2 cups cooked white rice

1 pound shrimp, peeled and deveined

1 cup mixed greens

(peas, carrots, corn, green beans)

1/2 onion, chopped

2 cloves garlic, minced

2 tablespoons vegetable oil

2 tablespoons soy sauce

1 tablespoon oyster sauce

Salt and pepper to taste

Green onions for garnish

Preparation

Heat vegetable oil in a large skillet over medium-high heat. Add chopped onions and minced garlic and cook until fragrant. Add the shrimp and cook until pink, about 23 minutes. Add the mixed vegetables and fry for another 23 minutes. Add the cooked white rice to the pan and stir to combine with the shrimp and vegetables. Add the soy sauce and oyster sauce and toss to evenly coat the rice and vegetables. Season with salt and pepper to taste. Serve hot, garnished with chopped green onions.

LENTIL AND VEGETABLE STEW

Preparation time: 45 minutes

Serves: 6 people

ingredients

1 cup dried lentils, rinsed and drained

2 cups vegetable broth

2 cups mixed greens

(carrots, celery, onions, potatoes)

2 cloves garlic, minced

2 tablespoons of olive oil

1 tablespoon of tomato paste

1 teaspoon dried thyme

1 bay leaf

Salt and pepper to taste

Fresh parsley for garnish

Preparation

Heat the olive oil in a large pot over medium-high heat. Add the minced garlic and cook until fragrant. Add the mixed vegetables and cook until they begin to soften, about 5 to 7 minutes. Add the rinsed and drained lentils, vegetable broth, tomato paste, thyme and bay leaf to the pan. Bring the mixture to the boil, then reduce the heat and simmer until the lentils are tender, about 30/40 minutes. Season with salt and pepper to taste. Serve hot, garnished with fresh parsley.

SWEET POTATO CHILI
AND BLACK BEANS

Preparation time: 45 minutes

Serves: 6 people

Ingredients:

2 medium sweet potatoes, peeled and cut into cubes

1 (15 ounce) can black beans, rinsed and drained

1 can (14.5 ounces) diced tomatoes

1 onion, chopped

3 cloves garlic, minced

2 tablespoons of olive oil

2 tablespoons chili powder

1 teaspoon ground cumin

1 teaspoon dried oregano

Salt and pepper to taste

Fresh coriander for garnish

Preparation

Heat the olive oil in a large pot over medium-high heat. Add the chopped onion and minced garlic and cook until the onion is translucent, about 5 minutes. Add the diced sweet potatoes, chili powder, cumin, and oregano to the pot and stir to combine. Add enough water to the pot to cover the sweet potatoes and bring to a boil. Reduce the heat and let the sweet potatoes simmer until tender, about 15 to 20 minutes. Add the rinsed and drained black beans and diced tomatoes to the pot and stir to combine. Let the chili simmer for another 10 to 15 minutes to allow the flavors to blend together. Season with salt and pepper to taste. Serve hot, garnished with fresh coriander.

TURKEY CHILI
AND VEGETABLES

Preparation time:

about 30/40 minutes

Serves 4:

ingredients

400 g turkey breast

1 hot pepper

2 courgettes

1 onion

2 ripe tomatoes

Salt to taste

Extra virgin olive oil to taste

Preparation

Dice the turkey breast and set aside. Slice the onion and sauté it in a pan with oil. Cut the courgettes into cubes and add them to the pan with the onion. Wash and dice the tomatoes and add them to the pan. Finely chop the chilli and add it to the pan. Season with salt and cook for about 10 minutes. In a separate pan, brown the turkey cubes with a drizzle of oil until golden brown. Add the turkey to the pan with the vegetables and cook for another 5 minutes. Serve hot.

BEAN AND VEGETABLE STEW

Preparation time: approximately 1
one hour and 30 minutes
For 4 people:
Ingredients:
400 g of cannellini beans
(or borlotti beans)
2 carrots, 2 celery
1 onion, 2 potatoes
2 ripe tomatoes
Vegetable broth to taste
Salt to taste
Extra virgin olive oil to taste

Preparation

Soak the beans in cold water overnight. Finely chop the onion and sauté it in a pan with oil. Dice the carrots, celery and potatoes and add them to the pot with the onion. Cut the tomatoes into cubes and add them to the pot. Season with salt and cook for about 10 minutes. Add the drained beans and vegetable broth until all the ingredients are covered. Cook over medium-low heat for about 1 hour, stirring occasionally, until the vegetables and beans are soft and the broth has reduced. Serve hot.

MINESTRONE WITH BARLEY AND BEANS

Preparation time: approximately 1 hour

Servings: 4

ingredients:

1 onion, diced

2 carrots, diced

2 stalks celery, diced

2 cloves garlic, minced

1 can diced tomatoes

1 can of red kidney beans, drained and rinsed

1 cup pearl barley

6 cups vegetable broth

1 teaspoon dried thyme

1 teaspoon dried basil

1 teaspoon dried oregano

Salt and pepper to taste

2 cups shredded cabbage

Preparation

In a large pot or Dutch oven, heat a drizzle of oil over medium heat. Add the onion, carrots, and celery and saute until the vegetables begin to soften, about 5 minutes. Add the garlic and cook for another minute. Add the diced tomatoes, beans, barley, vegetable broth, thyme, basil, oregano, salt and pepper. Bring to the boil. Reduce the heat to low and simmer for 45 minutes to 1 hour, or until the barley is tender. Add the shredded cabbage to the pot and stir until wilted, about 23 minutes. Serve hot, garnished with additional herbs, if desired.

LENTIL SOUP WITH CABBAGE AND TOMATOES

Preparation time:

approximately 45 minutes

Serves 4 people

ingredients

1 onion, chopped

2 carrots, diced

2 stalks celery, diced

2 cloves garlic, minced

1 cup dried lentils

4 cups vegetable broth

1 cup cherry tomatoes, cut in half

2 cups cabbage, chopped

1 teaspoon smoked paprika

Salt and pepper to taste

Extra virgin olive oil

Preparation

In a large pot or Dutch oven, heat a drizzle of oil over medium heat. Add the onion, carrots and celery and cook until the vegetables begin to soften about 5 minutes. Add the garlic and paprika and cook for another 2 minutes. Add the lentils and vegetable broth to the pot. Bring to the boil. Reduce the heat and simmer for about 25 to 30 minutes, or until the lentils are soft. Add the cherry tomatoes and shredded cabbage to the pot. Cook for an additional 5 minutes or until the cabbage is wilted. Season with salt and pepper to taste. Serve hot, garnished with a drizzle of extra virgin olive oil.

SPICY BLACK BEAN SOUP WITH CORN AND TOMATOES

Preparation time: approximately 45 minutes

Serves 4 people

ingredients

2 tablespoons extra virgin olive oil

1 onion, chopped

2 cloves garlic, minced

1 red chilli, chopped

2 cups canned black beans, rinsed and drained

1 cup canned sweet corn, rinsed and drained

2 cups peeled tomatoes, cut into pieces

4 cups vegetable broth

1 teaspoon ground cumin

1 teaspoon smoked paprika

Salt and pepper to taste

chopped fresh coriander (optional)

Preparation

In a large pot or Dutch oven, heat the oil over medium heat. Add the onion, garlic and chilli and cook until the vegetables begin to soften about 5 minutes. Add the black beans, corn, peeled tomatoes, vegetable broth, cumin, paprika and a little salt and pepper. Mix well and bring to the boil. Reduce the heat and simmer for about 20/25 minutes, or until the soup has become quite thick and creamy. Taste and adjust salt and pepper to taste. If you like, you can add chopped fresh coriander as a garnish. Spicy Black Bean Soup with Corn and Tomatoes is ready to enjoy! Serve hot with fresh bread or tortillas for a complete and tasty meal.

QUINOA AND VEGETABLE SOUP

Preparation time: approximately 45 minutes

Serves 4 people

Ingredients:

1 tablespoon extra virgin olive oil

1 onion, chopped

2 carrots, diced

2 stalks celery, diced

3 cloves garlic, minced

1 teaspoon turmeric powder

1 teaspoon cumin powder

1 cup quinoa, rinsed and drained

4 cups vegetable broth

2 cups fresh spinach, chopped

Salt and pepper to taste

chopped fresh coriander (optional)

Preparation

In a large pot or Dutch oven, heat the oil over medium heat. Add the onion, carrots, celery and garlic and cook until the vegetables begin to soften, about 5 to 7 minutes. Add the turmeric, cumin and quinoa and mix well to distribute the spices and lightly toast the quinoa. Add the vegetable broth and bring to the boil. Reduce the heat and simmer for about 20 to 25 minutes, or until the quinoa is cooked and the soup has become quite thick and creamy. Add the spinach and stir until wilted. Taste and adjust salt and pepper to taste. If you like, you can add chopped fresh coriander as a garnish. The quinoa and vegetable soup is ready to be enjoyed! Serve hot with fresh bread or croutons for a complete and healthy meal.

CHICKEN AND VEGETABLE SOUP WITH BARLEY

Preparation time: approximately 1 hour

Serves 4 people

Ingredients:

1 tablespoon extra virgin olive oil

1 onion, chopped

3 carrots, diced

2 stalks celery, diced

2 cloves garlic, minced

1 teaspoon dried thyme

1 teaspoon dried rosemary

1 cup pearl barley

4 cups chicken broth

2 cups of water

2 cups chicken breast, diced

2 cups fresh spinach, chopped

Salt and pepper to taste

grated parmesan (optional)

Preparation

In a large pot or Dutch oven, heat the oil over medium heat. Add the onion, carrots, celery and garlic and cook until the vegetables begin to soften, about 5 to 7 minutes. Add the thyme, rosemary and barley and mix well to distribute the spices and lightly toast the barley. Add the chicken stock and water and bring to a boil.

Reduce the heat and simmer for about 20 to 25 minutes, or until the orzo is cooked and the soup has become quite thick and creamy. Add the chicken and spinach and stir until the chicken is cooked and the spinach is wilted. Taste and adjust salt and pepper to taste. If you like, you can add some grated parmesan to garnish. Chicken and vegetable soup with barley is ready to enjoy! Serve hot with fresh bread or croutons for a complete and tasty meal.

SKEWERS GRILLED VEGETABLES WITH LEMON AND GARLIC

Preparation time:

about 30/40 minutes

Serves 4 people

Ingredients:

2 courgettes, diced

2 peppers, diced

1 red onion, diced

1 aubergine, diced

8 cherry tomatoes

1 lemon, juice and grated zest

2 cloves garlic, minced

2 tablespoons extra virgin olive oil

Salt and pepper to taste

8 skewers

Preparation

In a large bowl, whisk together the lemon juice, lemon zest, garlic, olive oil, salt, and pepper. Add the diced vegetables to the bowl and mix well to coat them with the marinade. Leave to rest for about 10/15 minutes. Thread them onto skewer sticks, alternating the ingredients. Heat grill or nonstick skillet over medium-high heat. Grill the vegetable skewers for about 2 to 3 minutes on each side until the vegetables are lightly charred and soft. Serve the grilled vegetable skewers piping hot, decorating with a few cherry tomatoes and a drizzle of extra virgin olive oil.

BAKED SWEET POTATOES WITH ROSEMARY AND GARLIC

Preparation time: approximately 15 minutes

Cooking time: approximately 30/40 minutes

Serves 4 people

Ingredients:

4 medium sweet potatoes, peeled and cut

into cubes of approximately 23 cm

23 sprigs of fresh rosemary, finely chopped

34 cloves garlic, finely chopped

3 tablespoons of extra virgin olive oil

Salt and pepper to taste.

Preparation

Preheat the oven to 200°C. In a large bowl, mix together the diced sweet potatoes, chopped rosemary, minced garlic, olive oil, salt and pepper. Toss well to coat the sweet potatoes with the spices and oil. Spread the sweet potatoes on a baking sheet, trying to arrange them in a single layer. Cook the sweet potatoes and cook for about 30/40 minutes, turning them every 10/15 minutes to ensure even cooking, until they are soft and lightly browned. Serve the baked sweet potatoes with rosemary and garlic piping hot, garnished with a few sprigs of fresh rosemary.

STEAMED BROCCOLI WITH LEMON AND PARMESAN

Preparation time: approximately 10/15 minutes

Cooking time: approximately 57 minutes

Serves 4 people

Ingredients:

2 medium broccoli, divided into florets

2 tablespoons unsalted butter, room temperature

1 clove garlic, finely chopped

1 lemon, grated zest and squeezed juice

1/4 grated parmesan

Salt and pepper to taste.

Preparation

Fill a large pot with 23 inches of water and bring it to a boil. Add the broccoli florets to the pot and cover it with a lid. Steam the broccoli for about 57 minutes, or until soft but still crunchy. Meanwhile, in a small skillet, melt the butter over medium heat. Add the minced garlic to the pan and cook for 12 minutes, until golden and fragrant. Add the grated lemon zest and lemon juice to the pan and stir well to combine. Drain the steamed broccoli and place it in a large bowl. Pour the lemon-garlic sauce over the broccoli and toss well to coat it with the sauce. Sprinkle the grated parmesan over the broccoli and mix gently. Add salt and pepper to taste and serve hot.

GRILLED COURGETTES WITH BALSAMIC VINEGAR GLAZE

Preparation time:

approximately 15 minutes

Servings: 4 people

Ingredients:

4 medium courgettes

2 tablespoons of olive oil

salt and freshly ground black pepper

2 tablespoons balsamic vinegar

1 tablespoon honey

Preparation

Preheat grill to medium-high heat. Trim the ends of the courgettes and then cut them diagonally into slices about half a centimeter thick. In a bowl, combine the olive oil, salt and pepper. Add the zucchini slices and toss to coat them well with the oil. Place the courgettes on the grill and cook them for 4/5 minutes per side, until they are tender and well marked by the grill. While the courgettes are cooking, prepare the glaze. In a small saucepan, combine the balsamic vinegar and honey. Bring to the boil over medium-low heat and cook for 12 minutes, until the glaze has thickened slightly. Remove the courgettes from the grill and place on a serving plate. Pour over the icing and serve warm or at room temperature.

SAUTEED SPINACH WITH GARLIC AND LEMON

Preparation time:

approximately 10 minutes

Cooking time 15 minutes

Serves 4 people

Ingredients:

450 g of fresh spinach

1 tablespoon olive oil

2 cloves garlic, finely chopped

juice of 1/2 lemon

salt and freshly ground black pepper

Preparation

Rinse the spinach in cold water and dry them with a clean cloth. Heat the olive oil in a large skillet over medium-high heat. Add the garlic and cook for about 1 minute, until golden and fragrant. Add the spinach to the skillet, a handful at a time, and toss gently with a spatula to appear even. Continue to cook the spinach, stirring occasionally, until completely wilted and soft, about 5 to 7 minutes. Squeeze the juice of half a lemon onto the spinach and mix well. Add salt and pepper to taste. Remove from the heat and transfer the spinach to a bowl or serving plate. Serve hot or at room temperature.

TURKEY LASAGNE WITH LEAN RICOTTA

Preparation time 30 minutes

Cooking time 40/45 minutes

portions: 4 people

Ingredients:

250 g of dry lasagne

400 g of minced turkey meat

500 ml of tomato puree

1 onion chopped

2 cloves garlic, minced

2 tablespoons olive oil, 1 egg

250 g of low-fat ricotta

100 g grated parmesan

salt and freshly ground black pepper

Preparation

Prepare the lasagna sheets following the instructions on the package. Drain and set aside. In a large skillet, heat the olive oil over medium heat. Add the onion and garlic and cook until soft and translucent. Add the turkey meat to the pan and cook until cooked through and browned. Add the tomato puree, salt and pepper to the pan and mix well. Let it cook for about 10/15 minutes. In a separate bowl, beat the egg and mix it with the ricotta and grated parmesan. Add salt and pepper to taste. In a baking dish, spread a layer of dry lasagna, then a layer of turkey meat and finally a layer of ricotta mixture. Repeat until all ingredients are used up, finishing with a layer of ricotta mixture. Cover the pan with aluminum foil and cook in a preheated oven at 180°C for about 30 minutes.

VEGETABLES LASAGNE WITH SPINACH, COURGETTES, AND AUBERGINES

Preparation time 30 minutes

Cooking time 40 minutes

Serving size: 4 people

Ingredients:

250 g of dry lasagne

200g of fresh spinach

2 medium courgettes, cut into cubes

1 aubergine, diced

1 onion, chopped

2 cloves garlic, minced

500 ml of tomato sauce

250 g of fresh ricotta

100 g grated parmesan

2 tablespoons of olive oil

salt and freshly ground black pepper

Preparation

Prepare the lasagna following the instructions on the package. Drain and set aside. In a skillet, heat the olive oil over medium heat. Add the onion and garlic and cook until soft and translucent. Add the aubergines and courgettes to the pan and cook until soft and golden. Add the spinach to the skillet and cook until wilted. Add salt and pepper to taste.

In a separate bowl, mix the ricotta with the grated parmesan, salt and pepper. In a baking dish, lay out a layer of dry lasagne, then a layer of vegetables and finally a layer of ricotta mixture. Repeat until all ingredients are used up, finishing with a layer of ricotta mixture. Cover the pan with aluminum foil and cook in a preheated oven at 180°C for about 30 minutes. Remove the film and continue cooking for another 10/15 minutes, until the surface is golden and crispy.

PUMPKIN LASAGNA WITH LEAN MOZZARELLA

Preparation time: 30 minutes

Cooking time 35 minutes

Serving size: 4 people

Ingredients:

250 g of dry lasagne

600 g of pumpkin,

peeled and cut into cubes

200 g lean mozzarella

cheese cut into cubes

1 onion, chopped

2 cloves garlic, minced

500 ml of tomato sauce

250 g of fresh ricotta

100 g grated parmesan

2 tablespoons of olive oil

salt and freshly ground black pepper

Preparation

Prepare the lasagna following the instructions on the package. Drain and set aside. In a skillet, heat the olive oil over medium heat. Add the onion and garlic and cook until soft and translucent. Add the squash to the pan and cook until soft and golden. In a separate bowl, mix the ricotta with the grated parmesan, salt and pepper.

In a baking dish, lay out a layer of dry lasagne, then a layer of pumpkin and mozzarella and finally a layer of ricotta mixture. Repeat until all ingredients are used up, finishing with a layer of ricotta mixture. Cover the pan with aluminum foil and cook in a preheated oven at 180°C for about 30 minutes. Remove the film and continue cooking for another 10/15 minutes, until the surface is golden and crispy.

GRILLED SALMON WITH LEMON AND AROMATIC HERBS

Preparation time:

approximately 20 minutes

Servings: 4 people

Ingredients:

4 fresh salmon fillets

juice of 1 lemon

2 tablespoons of olive oil

1 clove garlic, minced

1 teaspoon dried thyme

1 teaspoon dried rosemary

salt and freshly ground black pepper

Preparation

Turn on the grill and let it heat up. Mix the lemon juice, olive oil, chopped garlic, thyme, rosemary, salt and pepper in a bowl. Brush the salmon fillets with the lemon and aromatic herb mixture. Place the salmon fillets on the grill and cook for about 5/7 minutes per side, until they are cooked but still juicy inside. Serve the salmon piping hot, accompanied by a slice of lemon and some fresh herbs.

BAKED COD WITH TOMATO AND OLIVES SAUCE

Preparation time: 20 minutes

Cooking time 40 minutes

Serving size: 4 people

Ingredients:

4 cod fillets

500 g of peeled tomatoes

1 onion chopped

2 cloves garlic, minced

1 chopped chilli pepper

100 g of pitted black olives

2 tablespoons of olive oil

1 tablespoon red wine vinegar

salt and freshly ground black pepper

Preparation

Turn on the oven and heat it to 200°C. In a skillet, heat the olive oil over medium heat. Add the onion, garlic and chilli and cook until soft and translucent. Add the peeled tomatoes to the pan and cook until soft. Add red wine vinegar, black olives, salt and pepper and mix well. Arrange the cod fillets in a baking dish. Pour the tomato sauce over the cod. Cover the pan with aluminum foil and cook for about 30/40 minutes, until the cod is cooked and the tomato sauce is reduced and thick.

PACKED TILAPIA WITH LEMON AND CAPERS

Preparation time:

approximately 20 minutes

Serves: 4 people

Ingredients:

4 tilapia fillets

1 lemon cut into thin slices

2 tablespoons of capers

2 tablespoons of olive oil

salt and freshly ground

black pepper

Preparation

Turn on the grill and let it heat up. Brush the tilapia fillets with olive oil and sprinkle with salt and pepper. Wrap each tilapia fillet in a slice of lemon. Place the tilapia fillets on the grill and cook for about 4/5 minutes per side, until cooked and golden. Serve the tilapia piping hot, garnished with capers and a few slices of lemon.

TUNA SALAD WITH GREEK YOGURT AND AVOCADO

Preparation time: approximately 20 minutes

Serving size: 4 people

Ingredients:

2 cans of canned tuna

1 ripe avocado

1 red pepper cut into cubes

1 red onion cut into thin slices

1 head of lettuce

4 tablespoons of Greek yogurt

the juice of 1/2 lemon

2 tablespoons of olive oil

salt and freshly ground black pepper

Preparation

Cut the avocado into cubes and place it in a bowl. Add the tuna, pepper and onion. Add the lettuce to the bowl and mix gently. In another bowl, mix Greek yogurt, lemon juice, olive oil, salt and pepper to create the dressing. Pour the dressing over the tuna salad and mix well. Serve the salad cold.

PENNE WITH ROASTED TOMATOES GARLIC AND OLIVE OIL

Preparation time:

approximately 30 minutes

Serves 4 people

ingredients

500 g penne

500 g of cherry tomatoes

3 cloves garlic, minced

4 tablespoons of olive oil

1 bunch of fresh basil

salt and freshly ground black pepper

Preparation

Turn on the oven and heat it to 200°C. Cut the cherry tomatoes in half and place them in a baking dish. Add the garlic, olive oil, salt and pepper and mix well. Cook the cherry tomatoes in the oven for about 15/20 minutes, until they are soft and lightly golden. Cook the penne in a pan of salted water until al dente. Drain them and place them in a bowl. Add the roasted cherry tomatoes to the penne and mix well. Add the chopped fresh basil and mix again. Serve the penne piping hot.

PENNE WITH PESTO, TOMATOES AND PARMESAN

Preparation time: approximately 20 minutes

Serving size: 4 people

Ingredients:

500 g penne

1 cup fresh basil leaves

1 clove of garlic

1/2 cup grated parmesan

1/2 cup pine nuts

1/2 cup olive oil

1 cup cherry tomatoes cut in half

salt and freshly ground black pepper

Preparation

Cook the penne in a pan of salted water until al dente. Drain them and place them in a bowl. In a food processor, chop the basil, garlic, parmesan and pine nuts. Gradually add the olive oil, stirring until you obtain a smooth and creamy pesto. Pour the pesto over the penne and mix well. Add the cherry tomatoes and mix again. Season with salt and pepper and serve the penne piping hot.

PENNE WITH ROASTED VEGETABLES AND SKINNY FETA CHEESE

Preparation time:

approximately 30 minutes

Serves 4 people

Ingredients:

500 g penne

2 courgettes cut into cubes

2 red peppers cut into cubes

1 red onion, diced

2 tablespoons of olive oil

1 cup crumbled low-fat feta cheese

salt and black pepper

Preparation

Turn on the oven and heat it to 200°C. Place the courgettes, peppers and onion in a baking dish. Add the olive oil, salt and pepper and mix well. Cook the vegetables in the oven for about 20/25 minutes, until they are soft and lightly golden. Cook the penne in a pan of salted water until al dente. Drain them and place them in a bowl. Add the roasted vegetables to the penne and mix well. Add the crumbled feta and mix again. Serve the penne piping hot.

BLACK BEAN AND CORN SALAD WITH LIME SAUCE

Preparation time:

approximately 15 minutes

Servings: 4 people

Ingredients:

1 can of black beans (about 400 g)

1 can of corn (about 400 g)

1 red pepper cut into cubes

1 red onion diced

1 ripe avocado cut into cubes

1/4 cup chopped fresh cilantro

2 tablespoons of olive oil

2 tablespoons lime juice

1/2 teaspoon ground cumin

salt and freshly ground black pepper

Preparation

Rinse and drain the black beans and corn and place them in a large bowl along with the bell pepper, onion, avocado and cilantro. In another bowl, whisk together the olive oil, lime juice, and cumin. Add salt and pepper to taste. Pour the dressing into the bowl of black beans and corn and mix well. Serve the salad cold.

SOUTIE WITH LENTILS AND VEGETABLES

Preparation time:

about 45/50 minutes

Serves: 4 people

Ingredients:

1 cup dried lentils

2 tablespoons of olive oil

1 onion diced

2 carrots cut into cubes

2 celery sticks cut into cubes

2 cloves garlic, minced

1 bay leaf

4 cups vegetable broth or water

salt and freshly ground black pepper

Preparation

Rinse the lentils and place them in a pot with enough water to cover. Bring to the boil and let them cook for about 20 minutes until tender but not too soft. Drain them and set them aside. In a large pot, heat the olive oil over medium-high heat. Add the onion, carrots, celery and garlic. Cook, stirring occasionally, for about 10 minutes, until the vegetables are soft. Add the bay leaf and vegetable broth or water and bring to a boil. Reduce the heat and add the lentils. Let cook for about 15/20 minutes, until the liquid has reduced and the lentils are soft and tender. Add salt and pepper to taste. Serve the sautéed lentils and vegetables piping hot.

CHICKPEA AND VEGETABLE CURRY

Preparation time:

approximately 30 minutes

Serves 4 people

Ingredients:

1 onion

2 cloves of garlic

2 carrots

2 courgettes

1 red pepper

1 yellow pepper

400g canned chickpeas

400ml coconut milk

2 tablespoons curry powder

2 tablespoons of olive oil

Salt and pepper to taste.

Preparation

Dice the onion, garlic, carrots, courgettes and peppers. In a large pan, fry the onion and garlic in olive oil for a few minutes. Add the carrots and peppers and cook for 5/7 minutes. Add the drained and rinsed courgettes and chickpeas. Mix well and cook for another 5 minutes. Add the curry, salt and pepper, then pour in the coconut milk. Mix well and let cook for another 5/10 minutes until the sauce has thickened. Serve the curry hot accompanied by basmati rice or naan bread.

THREE BEAN SALAD WITH VINAIGRETTE DRESSING

Preparation time:

approximately 15 minutes

Serves 4 people

Ingredients:

400g canned black beans

400 g canned cannellini beans

400 g of canned borlotti beans

150g canned sweetcorn

1 red pepper

1 red onion

2 tablespoons chopped fresh coriander

2 tablespoons of olive oil

2 tablespoons red wine vinegar

the juice of 1 lime

Salt and pepper to taste.

Preparation

Drain and rinse the beans and corn and place in a large bowl. Dice the pepper and onion and add them to the bowl. Prepare the vinaigrette by mixing together olive oil, red wine vinegar, lime juice, chopped cilantro, salt and pepper. Pour the vinaigrette into the bowl and mix well. Let the salad rest in the refrigerator for at least 30 minutes before serving.

SPINACH AND FETA OMELETTE

Preparation 15 minutes

ingredients

for 2 people

4 eggs

100g of fresh spinach

50 g of feta cheese

1 clove of garlic

Olive oil

Salt and pepper

Preparation

Clean the spinach and cut them into small pieces. Chop the feta. In a non-stick pan, fry the garlic clove in a little olive oil. Add the spinach and cook for 5/7 minutes until wilted. In a bowl, beat the eggs with a pinch of salt and pepper. Add the feta to the pan with the spinach and mix well. Pour the beaten eggs into the pan and cook over medium-low heat for about 8/10 minutes until the omelette has solidified. Flip the omelette using a lid or plate and cook the other side for another 5/6 minutes. Serve hot or cold.

MUSHROOM AND SWISS CHEESE OMELETTE

Preparation 16 minutes

ingredients

for 4 people:

8 eggs

300 g of champignon mushrooms

100g Swiss cheese

1 clove of garlic

Olive oil

Salt and pepper

Preparation

Clean the mushrooms and cut them into thin slices. Grate the Swiss cheese. In a non-stick pan, fry the garlic clove in a little olive oil. Add the mushrooms and cook them for 8/10 minutes until they are soft and golden. In a bowl, beat the eggs with a pinch of salt and pepper. Add the grated cheese to the pan with the mushrooms and mix well. Pour the beaten eggs into the pan and cook over medium-low heat for about 8/10 minutes until the omelette has solidified. Flip the omelette using a lid or plate and cook the other side for another 5/6 minutes. Serve hot or cold.

WHITE WHITE OMELETTE WITH SKINNY CHEESE AND VEGETABLES

Preparation time:

about 20/25 minutes

Servings for 4

Ingredients:

16 egg whites

2 diced courgettes

2 diced red pepper

2 onion, chopped

1 clove garlic, minced

100 g of diced low-fat cheese

1 tablespoon olive oil

Salt and pepper to taste.

Preparation

In a nonstick skillet, heat the olive oil over medium heat. Add the onion and garlic and sauté until soft and translucent. Add the courgettes and pepper and cook for about 5 minutes, until soft. Add the egg whites, low-fat cheese, salt and pepper. Mix gently. Cook the omelette over medium/low heat for about 10 minutes or until golden brown on the bottom. Turn the omelette with the help of a plate or lid and cook for another 5/10 minutes, until golden and cooked.

GREEK OMELETTE WITH SPINACH, TOMATO AND FETA CHEESE

Preparation time

about 25/30 minutes

Serves 4

ingredients

8 eggs

200g of fresh spinach

2 diced tomatoes

100g crumbled feta

1 onion chopped

1 clove garlic, minced

1 tablespoon olive oil

Salt and pepper to taste.

Preparation

In a nonstick skillet, heat the olive oil over medium heat. Add the onion and garlic and sauté until soft and translucent. Add the spinach and cook for about 2/3 minutes, until wilted. Add the tomato and feta and mix gently. In a bowl, beat the eggs with salt and pepper. Add the eggs to the pan with the other ingredients and mix well. Cook the omelette over medium-low heat for about 10 minutes or until golden brown on the bottom. Turn the omelette with the help of a plate or lid and cook for another 5/10 minutes, until golden and cooked. Enjoy your meal!

BAKED SALMON
WITH VEGETABLES

Serves 4 people

Preparation time:

about 30/35 minutes

Ingredients:

4 fresh salmon fillets

1 diced red pepper

1 diced yellow pepper

1 diced red onion

2 diced courgettes

2 cloves garlic, minced

2 tablespoons of olive oil

Fresh lemon juice

Salt and pepper to taste

Chopped fresh parsley for garnish

Preparation

Preheat the oven to 200°C. In a bowl, mix the peppers, onion, zucchini, garlic, salt and pepper. Distribute the vegetables in a baking dish and place the salmon fillets on top. Season the salmon with lemon juice and olive oil. Bake in the preheated oven for about 15/20 minutes or until the salmon is cooked and the vegetables are soft. Garnish with chopped parsley and serve.

TUNA WITH GREEN SAUCES AND CHICKPEA PURE

Preparation time:

about 20/25 minutes.

Portions for 4 people

Ingredients:

4 fresh tuna fillets

400 g of boiled chickpeas

2 cloves garlic, minced

2 tablespoons of olive oil

2 tablespoons of water

1 bunch of fresh parsley

1 bunch of fresh basil

1 tablespoon capers

2 anchovy fillets

Salt and pepper to taste.

Preparation

In a blender, blend the chickpeas, garlic, olive oil, water, salt and pepper until smooth. In another bowl, mix the parsley, basil, capers, anchovies, salt and pepper to make the green sauces. Heat a non-stick pan over medium-high heat and cook the tuna fillets for 2/3 minutes per side or until they are golden on the outside and pink on the inside. Serve the tuna fillets accompanied by chickpea puree and green sauces.

RECIPES
SECOND DISHES

ROAST CHICKEN WITH POTATOES AND ROSEMARY

Cooking time: 35/40 minutes

Serves 4 people

Ingredients:

4 skinless chicken breasts

4 medium sized potatoes

1 tablespoon olive oil

2 cloves garlic, minced

1 teaspoon chopped rosemary

Salt and black pepper to taste

Preparation

Preheat the oven to 200°C. Cut the potatoes into cubes and place them in a baking dish together with the chicken. In a bowl, mix the olive oil, garlic, rosemary, salt and pepper. Pour the olive oil mixture over the chicken pieces and potatoes. Mix well to evenly distribute the seasoning. Cook for about 35/40 minutes or until the chicken is golden and cooked through. Serve hot.

CHICKEN AND POTATO STEW

Cooking time: 20/25 minutes

Serves 4:

Ingredients:

500 g chicken breast cut into cubes

4 medium sized potatoes cut into cubes

1 onion chopped

2 diced carrots

2 cups chicken broth

1 tablespoon olive oil

2 bay leaves

Salt and black pepper to taste.

Preparation

In a saucepan, fry the onion in olive oil. Add the chicken and sauté until golden brown. Add the potatoes, carrots, chicken broth, bay leaves, salt and pepper. Cover and bring to a boil. Reduce the heat and cook for about 20/25 minutes or until the potatoes and carrots are soft. Serve hot.

CHICKEN WITH ALMONDS AND SPINACH

Cooking time: 20/25 minutes

Serves 4:

4 skinless chicken breasts

1/2 cup almond flour

1/4 cup flour

1/2 teaspoon salt

1/4 teaspoon black pepper

1/4 teaspoon paprika

1/4 teaspoon garlic powder

2 tablespoons of olive oil

2 cloves garlic, minced

6 cups fresh spinach

1/4 cup sliced almonds

Preparation

In a bowl, mix the almond flour, flour, salt, black pepper, paprika and garlic powder. Dredge the chicken breasts in the almond-flour mixture and shake off the excess flour. In a nonstick skillet, heat the olive oil and garlic over medium heat. Add the chicken breasts and cook for 6/7 minutes per side or until golden brown and cooked through. Remove the chicken from the pan and set aside on a plate covered with aluminum foil. Add the spinach to the same pan and cook for 2 to 3 minutes or until wilted. Add the sliced almonds and cook for another 2/3 minutes or until they are lightly golden. Serve the chicken with spinach and sliced almonds on the side.

CHICKEN CURRY WITH VEGETABLES

Preparation time:

approximately 30 minutes

for 4 people

Ingredients:

500 g chicken breast cut into cubes

1 diced red pepper

1 diced yellow pepper

1 onion diced

2 diced carrots

1 cup fresh or frozen peas

1 can diced tomatoes

1 cup coconut milk

2 tablespoons of olive oil

2 tablespoons curry powder

Salt and black pepper to taste

Chopped fresh coriander to garnish

Preparation

In a large pan, heat the olive oil and fry the onion until translucent. Add the chicken and cook until browned. Add the peppers, carrots, peas and diced tomatoes and mix well. Add the curry powder and mix well until the vegetables and chicken are completely coated in the curry. Add the coconut milk and bring it to the boil. Lower the heat and cook for about 15/20 minutes until the vegetables are cooked. Season with salt and black pepper to taste. Serve hot garnished with chopped coriander.

LEMON CHICKEN
WITH ASPARAGUS

Preparation time: 10 minutes

Cooking time: 20 minutes

Servings: 4 people

Ingredients:

4 chicken breasts

2 tablespoons of olive oil

1 clove garlic, minced

1 lemon, grated zest and juice

1/2 cup chicken broth

1 bunch asparagus, cut into small pieces

Salt and pepper to taste.

Preparation

Preheat the oven to 200°C. In a large skillet, heat the olive oil over medium heat and add the minced garlic. Cook for a minute. Add the chicken breasts and cook for 5 minutes per side, until golden brown. Add the grated lemon zest, lemon juice and chicken broth. Bring to the boil, then reduce the heat and cook for 5 minutes. Add the asparagus and cook for another 5 minutes, until the chicken and asparagus are cooked. Serve hot.

GRILLED CHICKEN WITH ARTICHOKES AND TOMATOES

Preparation time: 10 minutes

Cooking time: 20 minutes

Portion: 4 people

Ingredients:

4 chicken breasts

1 jar of artichoke hearts,

drained and cut in half

1 cup cherry tomatoes

2 tablespoons of olive oil

Juice of 1/2 lemon

Salt and pepper to taste.

Preparation

Preheat grill to medium-high heat. Brush chicken breasts with olive oil and sprinkle with salt and pepper. Grill the chicken breasts for 6 to 7 minutes per side or until cooked through. Add the artichoke hearts and grilled cherry tomatoes and grill for another 5/7 minutes. Squeeze the juice of half a lemon onto the chicken breasts at the end of cooking. Serve hot.

CHICKEN CACCIATORA WITH CARROTS AND CELERY

Preparation time: approximately 20 minutes

Cooking time: approximately 45 minutes

for 4 people:

Ingredients:

4 chicken legs, 2 carrots

2 stalks of celery, 1 onion

2 cloves of garlic

2 tablespoons of tomato paste

1 glass of red wine

1 cup chicken broth

1 sprig of rosemary

Extra virgin olive oil

Salt and pepper

Preparation

In a large pan, heat the extra virgin olive oil. Add the chicken thighs and fry on both sides until golden brown. Remove the chicken thighs from the pan and set aside. In the same pan, add the diced onion, carrots and celery and sauté over medium heat for 5 minutes. Add the minced garlic and fry for another minute. Add the tomato puree and mix well. Pour the red wine into the pan and let it evaporate. Add the chicken broth and rosemary and bring to a boil. Return the chicken thighs to the pan and cover with the lid. Cook over medium-low heat for about 45 minutes or until the chicken is cooked through. Serve hot with white rice.

CHICKEN WITH PEPPERS AND COURGETTES

Preparation time: approximately 20 minutes

Cooking time: approximately 30 minutes

Ingredients for 4 people:

Ingredients:

4 chicken breasts

2 peppers (1 red and 1 yellow)

2 courgettes

2 cloves of garlic

2 tablespoons extra virgin olive oil

1 tablespoon dried oregano

Salt and pepper

Preparation

Preheat the oven to 200°C. Wash and cut the peppers into strips and the courgettes into slices. Arrange the vegetables in a baking dish and sprinkle them with extra virgin olive oil, salt, pepper and oregano. Mix the vegetables well and bake for 20 minutes. Meanwhile, in a large pan, heat a spoonful of extra virgin olive oil. Add chicken breasts and cook on both sides until browned. Add the minced garlic to the pan and fry for a minute. Remove the vegetables from the oven and distribute in the pan with the chicken. Mix everything well and cook for another 5/10 minutes. Serve hot.

PAPRIKA CHICKEN WITH ONIONS AND PEPPERS

Preparation: 15 minutes

Cooking time: 40 minutes

ingredients

for 4 people

4 chicken breasts

2 medium onions

2 red peppers

2 tablespoons of olive oil

2 tablespoons sweet paprika

1/2 teaspoon salt

1/4 teaspoon black pepper

1 cup chicken broth

Preparation

Cut the onions into thin slices and the peppers into strips. In a large skillet, heat the olive oil over medium-high heat and brown the chicken breasts until golden brown on both sides, about 5 to 7 minutes per side. Remove the chicken from the pan and set aside. Add the onions and peppers to the same pan and cook for about 5 minutes, until soft. Add the paprika, salt and black pepper and mix well. Add the chicken broth and boil for 12 minutes. Add the chicken to the pan and cover with the sauce. Reduce the heat and cook for about 20 to 25 minutes, or until the chicken is cooked.

TURKEY WITH GRILLED COURGETTES AND AUBERGINES

Preparation time:

about 30 minutes.

ingredients

portions for 4 people

4 slices of turkey breast

2 medium courgettes

1 large aubergine

1 clove of garlic

Extra virgin olive oil

Salt and pepper

Preparation

Cut the courgettes and aubergines into thin slices and grill them on a hot griddle or grill until soft and slightly charred. In a non-stick pan, brown the garlic clove with a drizzle of extra virgin olive oil. Add the turkey breast slices and cook until browned and cooked through. Add the grilled courgettes and aubergines to the pan with the turkey, along with a drizzle of extra virgin olive oil and a pinch of salt and pepper. Mix all the ingredients well and cook for 23 minutes so that the flavors blend. Serve the turkey with grilled courgettes and aubergines piping hot, accompanied by a side dish of seasonal vegetables or a mixed salad.

BAKED TURKEY
WITH VEGETABLES

Preparation time:

about 50 minutes

ingredients

for 4 people:

4 turkey breasts

2 courgettes

1 aubergine

1 pepper

1 onion

2 cloves of garlic

Olive oil to taste

Salt and pepper to taste

Preparation

Take a baking dish and arrange the turkey breasts. Cut the courgettes, aubergines and pepper into cubes and the onion into thin slices. Add the vegetables to the roasting pan with the turkey. Chop the garlic cloves and sprinkle them over the vegetables and turkey. Season with salt, pepper and olive oil. Cook in the oven at 180°C for approximately 40/45 minutes or until the turkey is cooked and the vegetables are soft. Serve hot.

BAKED SALMON
WITH ASPARAGUS

Preparation time:

approximately 25 minutes

ingredients

for 4 people:

4 salmon fillets of

approximately 150 g each

500 g of fresh asparagus

2 tablespoons of olive oil

Salt and pepper to taste

1 lemon

Preparation

Preheat the oven to 200°C. Wash the asparagus and cut the hard parts at the base. Place them in a baking dish and season them with a spoonful of extra virgin olive oil, salt and pepper. Mix well to distribute the seasoning. Cook the asparagus in the oven for about 10 minutes, until tender. In the meantime, wash the salmon fillets, dry them with absorbent paper and season them with salt, pepper and the juice of half a lemon. Transfer the salmon fillets to the pan with the asparagus and drizzle with a spoonful of olive oil. Cook for about 12/15 minutes, until the salmon is golden and cooked. Serve the salmon with asparagus and garnish with lemon slices.

GRILLED TUNA WITH TOMATOES AND CAPERS

preparation time 25 minutes

ingredients

for 4 people:

4 fresh tuna fillets

2 tablespoons of olive oil

1 clove of minced garlic

1 lemon (juice and grated zest)

1 cup cherry tomatoes cut in half

1 tablespoon capers

Salt and pepper to taste.

Preparation

Turn on the grill and brush with a little oil. In a bowl, mix the olive oil, minced garlic, lemon juice and zest. Brush the marinade over the tuna fillets and add salt and pepper to taste. Place the tuna on the grill and cook for 3/4 minutes per side, depending on the thickness of the fillet. In the meantime, in a pan over medium-high heat, brown the cherry tomatoes for 2/3 minutes, add the capers and cook for another 2/3 minutes. Serve the tuna with cherry tomatoes and capers as a side dish.

SEABASS IN PAPER WITH ARTICHOKES AND POTATOES

Preparation time 50 minutes

ingredients

for 4 people

4 sea bass fillets

4 artichokes

4 medium potatoes

2 cloves of garlic minced

1 lemon

1/2 glass of white wine

Olive oil to taste

Salt and pepper to taste.

Bay leaves to taste

Preparation

Preheat the oven to 200°C. Clean the artichokes and cut them into thin slices. Peel the potatoes and cut them into cubes. In a bowl, mix the artichokes, potatoes, garlic, lemon juice, olive oil, salt and pepper. Divide the vegetable mixture into 4 portions and place them in the center of 4 sheets of baking paper. Place a sea bass fillet on top of each mixed vegetable. Squeeze the lemon over the sea bass fillets, add a little salt and pepper, a spoonful of olive oil and a few bay leaves. Close the parcels and bake for about 20/25 minutes. Remove from the oven, open the foil and serve.

SHRIMP SKEWERS WITH COURGETTES AND TOMATOES

Serves 4 people

Preparation time: 20 minutes

Cooking time: 10/12 minutes

ingredients

500 g of peeled prawns

2 medium courgettes

250 g of cherry tomatoes

1 clove of garlic

2 tablespoons extra virgin olive oil

Salt and pepper to taste.

Preparation

Cut the courgettes into slices and wash the cherry tomatoes. Thread the prawns, courgette slices and cherry tomatoes onto the skewers, alternating. In a pan, fry the garlic with olive oil. Add the skewers and cook them over medium heat for 5/6 minutes per side. Season with salt and pepper to taste. serve hot.

BREAM FILLETS AL LEMON WITH ARTICHOKES AND ASPARAGUS SALAD

Serves 4 people

Preparation time: 20 minutes

Cooking time: 20/25 minutes

ingredients

4 sea bream fillets

8 artichokes

2 bunch of green asparagus

2 lemon

2 tablespoons extra virgin olive oil

Salt and pepper to taste.

Preparation

Clean the artichokes by removing the hard outer leaves and cutting them into wedges. Drain them for 10 minutes in boiling water and drain. Wash the asparagus and cut them into small pieces. Blanch them for 5 minutes in boiling water and drain them. Cut the lemon into thin slices. Place the sea bream fillets in a baking dish and sprinkle them with the juice of half a lemon, a pinch of salt and pepper. Place the artichokes and asparagus on top, add the lemon slices and olive oil. Cover the pan with baking paper and bake in a preheated oven at 180°C for 20/25 minutes. Serve the fish with the vegetables and season with the remaining lemon juice.

BAKED SOLE WITH ARTICHOKES AND PARSLEY

Preparation time: 20 minutes

Cooking time: 30 minutes

Serves 4:

4 sole

8 artichokes

1 clove of garlic

1 sprig of chopped parsley

Olive oil

Salt and pepper

Preparation

Clean the artichokes, remove the outer leaves, remove the tip and stem and cut them into segments. Place the artichokes in a bowl with water and lemon to prevent them from blackening. Rinse the sole, dry them with absorbent paper and salt them lightly. In a pan, fry the garlic with olive oil, add the artichokes and cook for 5/10 minutes until soft. Take a baking tray, grease it with oil and place the sole on it. Add the artichokes around the sole, sprinkle with chopped parsley, season with salt and pepper and drizzle with a drizzle of olive oil. Place the pan in a preheated oven at 180°C and cook for about 30 minutes, until the fish is golden and the artichokes are soft.

PEPPERS STUFFED WITH QUINOA AND VEGETABLES

Preparation time: 10 minutes

Cooking time: 30 minutes

for 4 people:

Ingredients:

4 large peppers

1 cup quinoa

2 cloves of garlic

1 courgette, 1 onion

1 carrot, 1 tomato

1 cup grated cheese

Olive oil

Salt and pepper to taste.

Preparation

Preheat the oven to 200°C. Wash the peppers, remove the caps and remove the seeds and internal filaments. In a saucepan, cook the quinoa according to the package directions. In a pan, heat the olive oil and fry the finely chopped onion and garlic. Add the diced carrot and courgette and the chopped tomato. Add the cooked quinoa to the vegetables and mix well. Season with salt and pepper to taste. Stuff the peppers with the quinoa and vegetable mixture. Arrange the peppers in a baking dish and sprinkle them with grated cheese. Cook for about 30 minutes, until the peppers are soft and the cheese is golden on top. Serve hot.

COURGETTES STUFFED WITH RICOTTA AND SPINACH

Preparation: about 20 minutes

Cooking: approximately 25 to 30 minutes

Servings: 4 servings

Ingredients:

4 courgettes

200g of fresh spinach

200 g of fresh ricotta

1 clove of garlic

50 g of grated parmesan

Extra virgin olive oil

Salt and pepper

Preparation

Preheat the oven to 180°C (350°F). Cut the courgettes in half lengthwise and empty them with a teaspoon. Chop the garlic and sauté it in a pan with extra virgin olive oil. Add the spinach to the pan and tilt. In a bowl mix the ricotta, grated parmesan, spinach and garlic. Season with salt and pepper. Stuff the courgettes with the mixture obtained. Place the stuffed courgettes in a baking tray and cook for about 25/30 minutes, until they are soft to the touch with a fork.

ARTICHOKES AND ONION OMELETTE

Preparation: about 20 minutes

Cooking: approximately 20/25 minutes

Servings: 4 servings

Ingredients:

6 eggs

2 artichokes

1 onion

2 tablespoons of oil

extra virgin olive oil

Salt and pepper

Preparation

Clean the artichokes, removing the outer leaves and thorns, until you obtain the heart. Cut them into thin slices. Chop the onion and fry it in a pan with extra virgin olive oil. Add the artichokes to the pan and cook until soft. In a bowl, beat the eggs with a pinch of salt and pepper. Add the artichokes and onion to the beaten eggs and mix well. Pour the mixture into the pan where you cooked the artichokes and cook over medium-low heat for about 10/12 minutes until cooked. Flip the omelette onto a plate and cook it on the other side for about 5/7 minutes. Serve hot.

**ASPARAGUS SALAD
WITH BOILED EGGS
AND ALMONDS**

Preparation time: 15 minutes

Cooking time 20 minutes

Servings: 4

ingredients:

450 gr. of asparagus, cut

and cut into 1-inch pieces

4 eggs, boiled and quartered

1/4 cup sliced almonds, toasted

2 tablespoons of olive oil

1 tablespoon white wine vinegar

1 teaspoon Dijon mustard

Salt and pepper to taste

Preparation

In a large pot of boiling salted water, blanch the asparagus for 23 minutes, until tender and crisp. Drain and rinse with cold water. In a small bowl, whisk together the olive oil, vinegar, mustard, salt, and pepper. In a large bowl, toss the asparagus with the dressing. Divide the asparagus among four plates and garnish with the hard-boiled eggs and toasted almonds.

ASPARAGUS AND RICOTTA PIE

Preparation time: 15 minutes

Cooking time: 40 minutes

Servings: 4

Ingredients:

1 pie crust (homemade or store-bought)

450 gr. Asparagus, cut into 1-inch pieces

1/2 cup ricotta

1/2 cup grated mozzarella

2 eggs, 1/4 cup milk, 1/4 teaspoon salt

1/4 teaspoon black pepper

1/4 grated parmesan

Preparation

Preheat oven to 375°F. Roll out pie crust and place in 9-inch pie pan. In a large pan of boiling salted water, blanch the asparagus for 2/3 minutes, until tender and crunchy. Drain and rinse with cold water. In a medium bowl, whisk together the ricotta, mozzarella, eggs, milk, salt and pepper. Arrange the asparagus in the tart and pour the ricotta mixture over it. Sprinkle the Parmesan cheese over the cake. Bake for 40 minutes, until the crust is golden and the filling is ready. Allow the cake to cool for a few minutes before slicing and serving.

GRATINATED CAULIFLOWER WITH TOMATO AND BASIL SAUCE

Preparation time 45/50 minutes, serves 4 people

Ingredients:

1 head of cauliflower, broken into florets

2 cups tomato sauce

1/4 cup fresh basil, chopped

1/2 cup grated parmesan

1/2 cup breadcrumbs

2 tablespoons of olive oil

Salt and pepper to taste

Preparation

Preheat the oven to 190°C. Steam the cauliflower florets for about 5 minutes or until tender. In a large bowl, combine the tomato sauce, chopped basil, salt and pepper. Mix well. Add the steamed cauliflower to the bowl and toss to coat. Transfer the mixture into a baking dish. In a separate bowl, combine the grated parmesan and breadcrumbs. Mix well. Sprinkle the breadcrumb mixture over the cauliflower mixture. Drizzle olive oil over the top. Bake in the preheated oven for about 20 to 25 minutes or until golden brown and crispy on top. Serve hot.

ROMAN-STYLE ARTICHOKES WITH POTATOES

Preparation time 10 minutes

Cooking time 45 minutes,

serves 4 people

Ingredients:

4 medium-sized artichokes

4 medium sized potatoes

1 lemon

1/4 cup olive oil

1/2 glass of water

Salt and pepper to taste

Preparation

Preheat the oven to 190°C. Wash the artichokes and remove the external leaves until you reach the tender internal leaves.

Cut off the top inch of each artichoke and cut off the stem. Cut the potatoes into wedges. In a bowl, combine the juice of one lemon, olive oil, salt and pepper. Mix well. Dip the artichokes and potatoes in the lemon and oil mixture. Arrange the vegetables in a baking dish. Add 1/2 cup water to the bottom of the dish. Cover the dish with aluminum foil. Cook in the preheated oven for approximately 45/50 minutes or until the artichokes and potatoes are tender. Remove the foil and cook for another 5/10 minutes or until the vegetables are golden on the surface. Serve hot.

BAKED ASPARAGUS WITH HAM AND CHEESE

Preparation time: 10 minutes

Cooking time: 25 minutes

Servings: 4

Ingredients:

450 gr. of asparagus, hard ends cut off

120 gr. of thinly sliced ham, chopped

100 gr. of grated cheddar cheese

50 gr. of grated parmesan

50 gr. cup of breadcrumbs

1 tablespoon olive oil

Salt and pepper to taste

Preparation

Preheat oven to 375°F. Arrange asparagus in a single layer in a baking dish. Pour the olive oil over the asparagus and season with salt and pepper. Sprinkle the ham over the asparagus. In a separate bowl, mix together the cheddar cheese, parmesan, and breadcrumbs. Sprinkle the cheese mixture over the ham and asparagus. Bake for 25 to 30 minutes or until cheese is melted and bubbly.

ASPARAGUS AND
BACON OMELETTE

Preparation time: 10 minutes

Cooking time: 15 minutes

Servings: 4

ingredients:

8 eggs

1 cup milk

450 gr. Asparagus cut into 1 inch pieces

8 slices bacon, chopped

100g grated cheddar cheese

Salt and pepper to taste

1 tablespoon butter

Preparation

In a bowl, whisk together the eggs and milk. Season with salt and pepper. In a large skillet, cook the bacon until crispy. Remove with a slotted spoon and set aside. Add the asparagus to the pan and cook for 3 to 4 minutes until tender. Remove from pan and set aside. Melt the butter in the pan over medium heat. Pour in the egg mixture and leave to cook for 2/3 minutes until the edges begin to set. Add the asparagus and bacon to half the omelette. Sprinkle with cheddar cheese. Using a spatula, fold the other half of the omelet over the filling. Cook for another 2/3 minutes until the cheese melts and the egg is cooked. Serve hot.

SLICED BEEF WITH ARUGULA AND TOMATOES

Preparation time 10 minutes

Cooking time 20 minutes

Serves: 4

Ingredients:

500 gr. Beef loin, thinly sliced

4 cups fresh arugula

1 cup cherry tomatoes, halved

2 tablespoons of olive oil

Salt and black pepper to taste

Preparation

Heat a large skillet over medium-high heat and add 1 tablespoon olive oil. Season the beef slices with salt and pepper, then add to the pan and cook for 3 to 5 minutes on each side, or until browned and cooked through. Remove the meat from the pan and set it aside to rest. In a large bowl, toss the arugula and cherry tomatoes with the remaining tablespoon of olive oil. Serve the meat on a tray or individual plates, topped with the rocket and tomato mixture.

BEEF STEW WITH POTATOES AND CARROTS

Preparation time: 20 minutes

Cooking time: 1 hour

Serves: 4

Ingredients:

600 gr. of beef stew meat, cut into 1-inch pieces

4 cups beef broth

2 cups of water

1 large onion, chopped

4 cloves garlic, minced

4 medium potatoes, peeled and cut into 1-inch pieces

4 medium carrots, peeled and
cut into 1-inch pieces

2 bay leaves

2 teaspoons dried thyme

Salt and black pepper to taste

Preparation

In a large pot or Dutch oven, heat 1 tablespoon olive oil over medium-high heat. Add the meat and cook until browned on all sides, about 5 minutes. Remove the meat from the pan and set it aside. Add the chopped onion to the pot and cook until softened, about 5 minutes. Add the minced garlic and cook for another minute.

Return the meat to the pot and add the beef broth, water, bay leaves, thyme, salt and pepper. Bring the mixture to a boil, then reduce the heat to low and simmer, covered, for 1 hour. Add the chopped potatoes and carrots to the pot and continue to simmer, covered, for another hour, or until the vegetables are tender and the meat is cooked through. Remove the bay leaves and serve the beef stew hot, garnished with chopped parsley if desired.

BEEF AND ASPARAGUS IN A PAN

Preparation time: 10 minutes

Cooking time: 15 minutes

Serves: 4

Ingredients:

500 gr. Beef loin, thinly sliced

1 bunch fresh asparagus, washed and cut into 2-inch pieces

2 cloves garlic, finely chopped

1 red chilli, finely chopped (optional)

2 tablespoons of olive oil

Salt and black pepper to taste

Juice of half a lemon

Chopped fresh parsley for garnish

Preparation

Heat the olive oil in a large skillet over medium-high heat. Add the minced garlic and chilli (if using) and sauté for about 1 minute. Add the sliced meat to the pan and cook for 2 to 3 minutes on each side, or until browned and cooked to your liking. Remove the meat from the pan and set it aside. Add the asparagus to the same pan and sauté for about 5/7 minutes, or until tender but still crunchy. Add the lemon juice to the pan and mix well. Return the meat to the pan and heat it for about 1/2 minute. Season with salt and black pepper to taste. Serve the beef and asparagus hot, garnished with chopped parsley.

ROAST BEEF WITH ARTICHOKES AND POTATOES

Preparation time: 20 minutes

Cooking time: 1 hour

Serves: 4

Ingredients:

500g of roast beef

100 gr. Of artichoke hearts, drained and quartered

4 medium potatoes, peeled and cut into small pieces

4 cloves garlic, minced

2 tablespoons of olive oil

2 teaspoons dried thyme

Salt and black pepper to taste

Preparation

Preheat the oven to 190°C. In a large baking dish, toss the potatoes, artichoke hearts, garlic, thyme, olive oil, salt, and black pepper until well coated. Place the beef roast on top of the vegetables in the roasting pan. Roast in the preheated oven for about 1 hour, or until the meat is cooked to your liking and the vegetables are tender and crisp. Let the meat rest for about 10 minutes before slicing. Serve the roast beef with the roasted artichokes and potatoes on the side.

BEEF MEATBALLS
WITH SPINACH

Preparation time: 20 minutes

Cooking time: 25 minutes

Serves: 4

Ingredients:

500 g of minced meat

1/2 cup breadcrumbs

1/4 cup milk

1 egg

2 cloves garlic, minced

1/4 grated parmesan

1/4 cup chopped fresh parsley

1/2 teaspoon salt

1/4 teaspoon black pepper

4 cups fresh spinach leaves

1 tablespoon olive oil

1 jar (24 ounces) marinara sauce

Shaved parmesan for garnish

Preparation

Preheat the oven to 200°C. In a large bowl, mix together the ground beef, breadcrumbs, milk, egg, garlic, grated Parmesan, chopped parsley, salt and black pepper until well combined. Using your hands, shape the mixture into 16 meatballs. Heat the olive oil in a large oven-safe skillet over medium-high heat.

Add the meatballs to the pan and cook for about 5 to 7 minutes, or until golden brown on all sides. Remove the pan from the heat and add the spinach leaves on top of the meatballs. Pour the marinara sauce over the spinach and meatballs. Bake in the preheated oven for about 20/25 minutes, or until the meatballs are cooked and the spinach is wilted. Serve hot, garnished with flakes of parmesan.

PORK CHOPS WITH APPLES AND POTATOES

Preparation time: 20 minutes

Cooking time: 60 minutes

Serves: 4

Ingredients:

700 gr. Pork ribs, cut into serving pieces

4 medium potatoes, peeled and cut into chunks

3 medium apples, cored and cut into pieces

1 large onion, chopped

2 cloves garlic, minced

1/4 cup olive oil

1/4 cup apple cider vinegar

1 tablespoon brown sugar

1 tablespoon dried thyme

Salt and black pepper to taste

Preparation

Preheat the oven to 175°C. In a large bowl, whisk together the olive oil, apple cider vinegar, brown sugar, dried thyme, salt, and black pepper. Add the pork ribs to the bowl and toss to coat well with the marinade. In a large baking dish, layer the chopped onion, potatoes and apples. Place the marinated pork ribs on top of the vegetables in the baking dish. Cover the baking sheet tightly with foil.

Roast in the preheated oven for about 1 hour and 30 minutes, or until the pork is cooked through and tender. Remove the foil from the pan and bake for a further 10 to 15 minutes, or until the pork is golden and crispy. Let the pork rest for about 5 minutes before serving. Serve hot, with roast potatoes and apples on the side.

ROAST PORK WITH PLUM AND CARROTS

Preparation time: 15 minutes

Cooking time: 60 minutes

Serves: 4

Ingredients:

700 gr. of boneless pork loin

Salt and black pepper to taste

1 tablespoon olive oil

1 onion, chopped

3 cloves garlic, minced

1 cup pitted plums

1 cup chicken broth

1/4 cup honey

2 tablespoons Dijon mustard

1 pound carrots, peeled and cut into pieces

Preparation

Preheat the oven to 190°C. Season the pork loin with salt and black pepper on all sides. Heat the olive oil in a large oven-safe skillet over medium-high heat. Add the pork loin to the pan and cook for about 5 minutes or until browned on all sides. Remove the pork from the pan and set aside on a plate. Add the chopped onion and minced garlic to the pan and sauté for about 23 minutes, or until the onion is translucent.

Add the pitted plums, chicken broth, honey, and Dijon mustard to the pan and stir to combine. Return the pork loin to the pan and pour the sauce over the pork. Add the carrot pieces to the pan around the pork loin. Roast in the preheated oven for about 1 hour, or until the pork is cooked through and tender. Let the pork rest for about 5/10 minutes before slicing it. Serve hot, garnished with chopped fresh parsley if desired.

PORK SKEWERS WITH GRILLED VEGETABLES

Preparation time: 20 minutes

Cooking time: 15 minutes

Serves: 4

Ingredients:

450 gr. Pork Tenderloin,

cut into 1-inch cubes

Salt and black pepper to taste

1/4 cup olive oil

2 tablespoons balsamic vinegar

1 tablespoon honey

1 tablespoon Dijon mustard

2 cloves garlic, minced

1 red pepper, seeded and cut into pieces

1 yellow pepper, seeded and cut into pieces

1 courgette, cut into pieces

1 red onion, chopped

8 wooden skewers, soaked in water for at least 30 minutes

Preparation

Pre Heat a grill or grill pan over medium/high heat. Season the pork cubes with salt and black pepper on all sides. In a small bowl, whisk together the olive oil, balsamic vinegar, honey, Dijon mustard, and minced garlic.

Thread the seasoned pork cubes onto the soaked wooden skewers, alternating with the pieces of peppers, courgettes and red onion. Brush the skewers with the marinade on all sides. Grill the skewers on the preheated grill or grill pan for about 10 to 15 minutes, or until the pork is cooked through and the vegetables are charred and tender. Serve hot, garnished with chopped fresh parsley or cilantro if desired.

PORK FILLET WITH MUSTARD AND HONEY SAUCE

Preparation time: 15 minutes

Cooking time: 25 minutes

Total time: 40 minutes

Serves: 4

Ingredients:

4 pork fillet, salt and pepper

2 tablespoons of olive oil

2 tablespoons Dijon mustard

2 tablespoons honey

1 tablespoon soy sauce

1/4 cup chicken broth

1/4 cup heavy cream

Preparation

Preheat the oven to 200°C. Season the pork fillets with salt and pepper. Heat the olive oil in a large skillet over medium-high heat. Add the pork fillets and cook for 2/3 minutes on each side until golden brown. Transfer the pork tenderloins to a baking dish. In a small bowl, whisk together the Dijon mustard, honey, soy sauce, and chicken broth. Pour the mustard mixture over the pork tenderloins. Cook for 15 to 20 minutes, or until the pork tenderloins are cooked. Transfer the pork tenderloins to a serving plate. Pour the cream into the pan and stir to combine with the mustard sauce. Cook for another 2/3 minutes or until the sauce has thickened. Pour the sauce over the pork fillets and serve.

SIDE DISH RECIPES

SPINACH AND STRAWBERRY SALAD

Preparation Times: 15 minutes

Cooking Times: 0 minutes

Doses for 4 People:

Ingredients:

Fresh spinach: 200 g

Strawberries: 200 g

Feta: 100 g

Shelled walnuts: 50 g

Balsamic vinegar: 2 tablespoons

Extra virgin olive oil: to taste

Salt to taste

Pepper as needed

Preparation:

Wash the spinach well and dry them. Wash the strawberries, remove the stems and cut them into slices. Crumble the feta. Shell the walnuts and chop them coarsely. In a large bowl, combine the spinach, strawberries, feta, walnuts, balsamic vinegar, oil, salt and pepper. Mix well and serve immediately.

GRILLED VEGETABLES

Preparation Times: 10 minutes

Cooking Times: 20 minutes

Doses for 4 People:

Ingredients:

Peppers: 2 (about 400 g)

Eggplant: 1 (about 300 g)

Courgette: 1 (about 200 g)

Onion: 1 (about 100 g)

Extra virgin olive oil: to taste

Salt to taste

Pepper as needed

Note:

Preparation

Wash the vegetables and cut them into similar sized pieces. Arrange the vegetables on a baking tray lined with baking paper. Drizzle with oil, salt and pepper. Bake in a preheated oven at 200°C for 20 minutes, or until the vegetables are golden and tender. For the grilled vegetables, you can use any type of vegetable you prefer. Grilled vegetables can be served hot or cold, as a side dish or as a main course.

QUINOA WITH VEGETABLES

Preparation time: 20 minutes

Cooking time: 20 minutes

Doses for 4 People:

Ingredients

200 g of quinoa

400 g of mixed vegetables (for example, courgettes, peppers, aubergines, onions)

2 tablespoons of extra virgin olive oil

1 clove of garlic

salt to taste

pepper to taste

Fresh basil (optional)

Preparation:

Wash the quinoa under running water to remove the saponin. In a pot, cook the quinoa in boiling water for about 15 minutes, or until tender. In the meantime, wash the vegetables and cut them into small pieces. In a pan, heat the olive oil and fry the garlic for a minute. Add the vegetables and cook for about 10 minutes, or until tender. Salt and pepper to taste. Drain the quinoa and add it to the cooked vegetables. Mix well and serve with fresh basil, if desired.

STEAMED GREEN BEANS WITH TOASTED ALMONDS

Preparation time: 10 minutes

Cooking time: 10 minutes

Doses for 4 People:

Ingredients

400 g of green beans

50 g of shelled almonds

2 tablespoons of extra virgin olive oil

1 tablespoon lemon juice

salt to taste

pepper to taste

Preparation:

Wash the green beans and cut the ends. Steam the green beans for about 10 minutes, or until tender. Meanwhile, toast the almonds in a non-stick pan for a couple of minutes, or until they are golden. In a bowl, combine the cooked green beans, toasted almonds, olive oil, lemon juice, salt and pepper. Mix well and serve.

Tips: For a more intense flavor, you can marinate the vegetables before cooking them. You can use any type of vegetable you like for quinoa. You can add other ingredients to the toasted almonds, such as raisins or pine nuts. Steamed green beans with toasted almonds served as a side dish.

CUCUMBER AND TOMATOES SALAD

Preparation time: 15 minutes

Cooking time: 0 minutes

Doses for 4 People:

Ingredients

2 medium cucumbers (about 400 g)

4 medium tomatoes (about 500 g)

1 medium red onion (about 150 g)

1/4 cup (60 ml) extra virgin olive oil

2 tablespoons (30 ml) fresh lemon juice

1 tablespoon (15 ml) balsamic vinegar

1/2 teaspoon fine salt

1/4 teaspoon ground black pepper

1/4 cup (60 g) crumbled feta (optional)

1/4 cup (60 g) pitted black olives (optional)

Preparation:

Wash the cucumbers, tomatoes and red onion thoroughly. Dry the vegetables well with a clean cloth. Cut the cucumbers in half lengthwise and then into thin slices. Cut the tomatoes in half and then into thin slices, removing the seeds. Finely slice the red onion. In a large bowl, combine the cucumbers, tomatoes and red onion. Season with extra virgin olive oil, lemon juice, balsamic vinegar, salt and pepper.

Stir gently to mix the seasoning well. Add crumbled feta and black olives, if desired. Mix again and serve the fresh salad.

Advice:

For a more intense flavor, you can add chopped fresh herbs, such as basil, mint or oregano, to the salad.

SAUTÉED   BROCCOLI WITH

GARLIC AND LEMON

Preparation Times: 15 minutes

Cooking Times: 10 minutes

Doses for 4 People:

Ingredients:

1 Broccoli: 500 g

Garlic: 8 g

Fresh lemon juice: 15 ml

Extra virgin olive oil: 20 g

Salt to taste

Pepper as needed

Preparation:

Wash the broccoli carefully and cut it into florets. In a large pan, heat the extra virgin olive oil and fry the garlic until golden. Add the broccoli florets and cook for about 5 minutes, stirring occasionally. Add the lemon juice and cook for another 5 minutes, or until the broccoli is tender. Salt and pepper to taste. Serve the sautéed broccoli with hot garlic and lemon.

Advice:

For a more intense flavor, you can add a pinch of chili powder to the broccoli during cooking. Broccoli sautéed with garlic and lemon can be enriched with other ingredients, such as crispy bacon, toasted pine nuts or salted ricotta. This dish is an excellent source of vitamins and minerals.

GRILLED ASPARAGUS WITH LEMON AND PARMESAN

Preparation Time: 10 minutes

Cooking time: 10 minutes

Doses for: 4 people

Ingredients:

500g asparagus, washed and ends split

2 tablespoons of olive oil

Grated zest of 1 lemon

Juice of 1/2 lemon

Salt to taste

Pepper as needed

Grated Parmesan for garnish

Thin lemon slices for decoration (optional)

Chopped fresh parsley for garnish (optional)

Preparation:

1. Prepare the Asparagus: Wash the asparagus and cut the tough ends. 2. Marinate the Asparagus: In a large bowl, toss the asparagus with the olive oil, grated lemon zest, lemon juice, salt and pepper. Make sure the asparagus is evenly coated. 3. Grill the Asparagus: Heat a grill or nonstick pan over medium-high heat. Place the asparagus on the grill and cook for about 45 minutes per side, turning once, until tender and lightly browned.

4. Complete the Dish: Transfer the grilled asparagus to a serving platter. **5. Garnish and Serve:** Sprinkle the asparagus with plenty of grated Parmesan cheese. If desired, decorate with thin slices of lemon and chopped fresh parsley. Serve the grilled asparagus hot as an elegant and tasty side dish

CONCLUSION

Thank you for taking this journey with us through the world of the DASH Diet. We hope this book has given you not only the knowledge you need to improve your health, but also the inspiration to embrace a healthier, more balanced lifestyle. The DASH Diet is not just a diet; it's a real lifestyle that can transform your physical and mental well-being. Through the chapters of this book, we have explored the scientific benefits of the DASH Diet, offered practical tools for meal planning, and shared delicious and nutritious recipes. We hope these resources have made it easier for you to adopt the DASH Diet into your daily routine and have motivated you to make healthy choices for you and your family.

Remember, every small step towards better nutrition is a big step towards a healthier life.

Consistency is the key to success and every positive change, no matter how small, can have a big impact in the long run. Don't forget to listen to your body, exercise regularly and maintain a balance between mind and body. We invite you to share your experience with the DASH Diet. Your reviews and feedback are extremely valuable to us and other readers.

If you found this book helpful, please leave a review and tell us how the DASH Diet has affected your life. Your words can inspire others to take the same path to better health. Thank you again for choosing "DASH 2025 Diet" to guide you on your journey to wellness. We wish you health, happiness, and continued success in your adventure with the DASH Diet. With gratitude,

[KLARLOCK]